Lord Liu Chun's Secrets of Longevity

Lord Liu Chun's Secrets of Longevity:

600 Years of Proven Cures

BERNARD HO

AND

ALETA LEE

iUniverse, Inc.
New York   Bloomington

Lord Liu Chun's Secrets of Longevity
600 Years of Proven Cures

iUniverse books may be ordered through booksellers or by contacting:

iUniverse
1663 Liberty Drive
Bloomington, IN 47403
www.iuniverse.com
1-800-Authors (1-800-288-4677)

ISBN: 978-1-4502-3532-7 (sc)
ISBN: 978-1-4502-3535-8 (ebook)
ISBN: 978-1-4502-3534-1 (dj)

Library of Congress Control Number 2010908429

Printed in the United States of America

iUniverse rev. date: 12/17/2010

To the past nine hundred years and to the future, as we try to live each day mindful of the words of Dr. Liu Wansu: "Do not seek to know one's future, but do good deeds."

And to my five children, Gabriel, Miki, Bernice, Bernadette and Gregory: Remember that there is much to be learned out there, from all over the world, and one must strive to keep an open mind.

Contents

Disclaimer

The information contained in this book is provided for your general information only. The authors of this book do not give medical advice or engage in the practice of medicine. This book does not make diagnoses, suggest treatment, or prescribe medications. The information is intended as an educational service to assist you in your personal research on certain medical topics. The authors provide no warranty, expressed or implied, as to the accuracy, reliability, or completeness of furnished data. No independent clinical trials were made to confirm the efficacies of the studies presented. All English/ Latin translations of herb names should be based on Chinese Medical Terminology.

Preface

I was able to compose *Lord Liu Chun's Secrets of Longevity: 600 Years of Proven Cures*, which presents research that Lord Liu Chun conducted six hundred years ago in English for the first time, thanks to three books by Dr. Liu Hong Zhang, Lord Liu's twenty-fourth-generation descendant.

For centuries, the Liu family has guarded the secrets Lord Liu discovered about healthy living and disease prevention through experiments he conducted in order to ascertain the most effective treatment of a wide range of diseases and health issues. Recently, Dr. Liu Hong Zhang published a portion of these family secrets in three tomes—*Lord Liu Chun's Enhancement of Life* (China Friendship Publisher, April 2006), which links food therapy and healthy living to the prevention of many diseases; *Your Lifestyle is the Cause of Disease* (August 2006), which details the effects of certain lifestyles that cause disease; *and Beware of Medicine* (February 2007), which discusses how medicine can cause new problem.

Dr. Liu wrote the books despite opposition from family members who didn't want him to reveal the secrets. His vision was to share the family's wealth of knowledge, and the three books disclose a tenth of Lord Liu's research.

The words of Lord Liu Chun and his twenty-fourth-generation descendent, as well as the Liu family recipes, formulae, and history that appear in *Lord Liu Chun's Secrets of Longevity* are taken from these three books. In addition, as I was writing this book, I e-mailed

Dr. Liu nearly every week for approximately two years, and I stayed in his house in China four times in order to learn directly from him.

My wife, Aleta Lee, helped me write the book. In addition, Traditional Chinese Medicine doctor Tu Hoa of Los Angeles was of great help. I sought his advice on Chinese herbs and methodology.

Lord Liu Chun's Secrets of Longevity covers only a portion of Dr. Liu's books.

After subtracting expenses and a reserve for the publication of the next book, Aleta and I would like to contribute all profits to charitable organizations.

Acknowledgments by Bernard Ho

The selfless efforts of many individuals helped to complete this book, and I would like to acknowledge some of the key contributors. First and foremost, I would like to thank Dr. Liu Hong Zhang and his son, Mr. Liu Bo, for their blessings and encouragement during the research and writing. Thank you for sharing with the world your many lessons and recipes aimed at helping us achieve a healthier lifestyle.

To Dr. Tu Hoa, in Los Angeles, thank you for your special contributions and expertise in traditional Chinese medicine and documentation.

To Mr. Zhao Ying Jian, writer and director, thank you for your help with conducting surveys all over China and for sharing the stories of patients who caregivers have successfully treated using Lord Liu Chun's formulae for liver problems, kidney failures, heart disease, and cancer.

To my friends and family, especially Dewy Ip, Patrick Ho, Chloe Ho, and Stephen Law, thank you for your financial support and enthusiasm for this project. This has been a group effort, and I could not have finished without your help.

To Inge Ho, thank you very much for your creativity and for designing the cover illustration.

To Aleta Lee, my wife, thank you for coauthoring this book and editing. Also, thank you for supporting me through many long days and for remaining a driving force on this project.

Chapter 1
The Last Request of Empress Yong Le

In 1407, Lord Liu Chun (刘纯侯爵) sat in his study and quietly contemplated his imminent death. Under his care, his cousin, Empress Yong Le (永乐皇后徐仪华), had died of breast cancer. He expected the emperor's decree to arrive at his home in Nanjing within the hour, and he knew it would order his execution.

He hoped the emperor would be lenient and spare the rest of his family. As head of the Imperial Physicians, a post he had held for six years, he had explored all possible avenues in his effort to cure the empress. He knew that the Ming emperor cherished his wife, a wise and benevolent ruler. She had been well-loved by her subordinates. Lord Liu Chun sat through his last night, waiting for the order to come.

Finally, the imperial eunuch arrived with the sentence from the emperor. Lord Liu Chun knelt to hear the decree, but there was only silence. After some time, the eunuch asked Lord Liu Chun to rise. Lord Liu Chun was very surprised and touched, as he remembered the old days when he had served his cousin, the empress, and when he had assisted the emperor in his ascension to the throne. Perhaps these actions would now sway the emperor toward a lenient decision.

The empress's last order had called for Lord Liu Chun to develop a cure for many diseases, including cancer. He was to perform experiments on death row prisoners. The emperor was to assign three hundred medical doctors and a few thousand soldiers to Lord Liu Chun's research team.

When Lord Liu Chun recovered from his shock, he immediately began to ponder how he was going to honor the empress's last request.

After careful consideration, he sought out the emperor's advisor, a well-known Buddhist monk (姚广孝僧人). At the monk's request, the emperor gave Lord Liu Chun a special seal from the Yuan dynasty (元朝) that had symbolized power and had represented the red Buddhist sect (花教). As a devout Buddhist, Lord Liu Chun requested that any prisoners who were cured during the experiments would be absolved of their crimes and released to the boundaries of China. In this way, many prisoners were given a second chance to live as free men.

For sixty-six years after the empress's death, Lord Liu Chun performed thousands of experiments and found many miraculous cures. He fulfilled the last wish of the dying empress.

Lord Liu Chun, the patron saint of Chinese Imperial Physicians during the Ming and Qing dynasties, was born in Hubei province in 1363 AD and lived to be 126 years old. In 1475, when he was 112 years old, he formulated his treatment plans for cancer, cardiovascular disease, diabetes, and mental illness through food therapy and lifestyle maintenance. He pioneered the use of bovine flexor tendon to inhibit the spread of cancer and shark gallbladder to treat cancer. He discovered that porcine and bovine skins were elemental in the treatment of lung and heart disease, diabetes, and mental illness. Through his comprehensive research, he identified the use of liver and blood from pig, cow, duck, and chicken to treat anemia. Lord Liu Chun also developed the key to good health: an appetite-inducing soup, which would stimulate true hunger and metabolism.

In the last six hundred years, the doctor descendants of Lord Liu and the Imperial Physicians of China have healed more than ten million patients. Lord Liu's path to health and longevity is predicated on the concept of balance between prevention and cure. Lord Liu described his treatment as:

七分养，三分治 (Seven parts nurturing, three parts healing)

The concept of food as medicine is an ancient one. Hippocrates, the founding father of Western medicine, wrote, "Thy food is thy medicine." Six hundred years ago, Lord Liu identified the use of liver and blood from pig, cow, duck, and chicken to treat anemia. In Western medicine, liver therapy and, more importantly, food therapy have played an important role in the study of health. In 1934, George H. Whipple, George R. Minot, and William P. Murphy received the Nobel Prize in medicine for their research on the use of liver therapy to treat pernicious anemia.

In the years before 1926, pernicious anemia was a common disease in the United States that claimed the lives of about six thousand people annually. Thus, we can estimate that between 1926 (when the liver therapy was first applied) and 1934 (when the Nobel Prize was awarded), up to twenty thousand people in the United States alone avoided death through the use of food as medicine.[1]

One of the oldest Chinese medical manuscripts, the *Huangdi Nei Jing* (皇帝内经), compiled in 400 BC, describes a good doctor as one who treats disease before the symptoms appear and a mediocre doctor as one who treats disease after the patient falls ill.

In our modern world, health care is one of the most costly items on the national budgets of industrialized countries. In 2008, total health care expenditures in the United States were over $2 trillion, representing 16.2 percent of the national budget.[2] By shifting to a preventive approach to medicine from a curative one, a government could simultaneously reduce its health care bill, improve productivity in the workplace, and increase the longevity of its citizens. To quote Tommy Thompson, former governor of Wisconsin, former secretary of the US Department of Health and Human Services, and national policy advisor for US Preventive Medicine, "The Prevention Plan could be the biggest innovation in health care in the last thirty years."[3]

Comparing Western and Chinese medical approaches, it would be reasonable to conclude that Western medical treatments excel in areas of disease analysis, surgical procedures, and emergency and immunization services. However, Chinese methods are very effective in the treatment of chronic diseases such as cancer, high blood pressure, diabetes, and hepatitis, since chronic diseases require, first and foremost, the enhancement of life.

Six hundred years ago, Lord Liu Chun documented his findings from thousands of experiments conducted over a span of sixty-six years. Amazingly, after six centuries, most of these theories continue to be accurate and relevant! During our research, we also found discrepancies between Lord Liu Chun's findings and modern research. These disagreements are important to the continual study of the possibilities of alternative medicine. Furthermore, there are many facets of Lord Liu Chun's treatments that have yet to be tested. Western research on the medical effects of squalamine, collagen type 1, elastin—most of the Western medical research correlating to Dr. Liu's practice presented in this book—dates back only twenty years. We could find very little relevant research regarding the issues we addressed dating further back. For everyone, regardless of his or her beliefs about which medical practices are best, exploring a healthy lifestyle and different methods to obtain it is a compelling and worthwhile effort.

Chapter 2
Sixty-Six Years of Experimentation

Lord Liu Chun spent two years discussing and planning the experimentation with his colleagues, three hundred medical doctors who the emperor had assigned to him. Lord Liu also received the assistance of several thousand soldiers from the Imperial Army. The emperor funded all his research.

Lord Liu collected 2,000 years of medical history, classified 2,175 diseases, and listed more than 5,000 types of herbs and ingredients and 61,739 recipes and formulae. His first step was to organize the diseases in sixteen classifications[i] (证候群). He created two more categories based on lack of hunger and appetite and proper consumption of food. He divided his staff into eighteen teams to study the eighteen classifications. The team conducted these experiments repeatedly over a span of several years.

At the same time, Lord Liu Chun tested each of the 5,611 herbs to identify their best applications. He conducted the experiments, which required the participation of hundreds of thousands of death row inmates, over a period of sixty-six years.

---

i   The sixteen classifications are difficult to translate. These classifications relate to the concept of pathogenic wind, pathogenic cold, pathogenic heat (fire), pathogenic dampness, and pathogenic dryness. The seven emotions, phlegm, blood stasis, and the imbalance of yin and yang also come into play. In *Lord Liu Chun's Secrets of Longevity*, I touch on only five of these classifications. I will address the concept in more detail in the book's sequel.

Lord Liu's family and the Imperial Physicians kept the results secret. Only in recent years has his twenty-fourth generation descendant, Dr. Liu Hong Zhang, revealed these secrets.

In 1409, five thousand death row inmates lived in Nanjing, and Lord Liu began eighteen simultaneous experiments. Lord Liu used all five thousand prisoners; he initially assigned three thousand six hundred people (eighteen groups of two hundred people each) for research. In the process of inducing illness in patients, some patients died prematurely; the researchers replaced them from the remaining inmates. Additionally, some patients did not become sick because of genetic predispositions, and the team also replaced those patients.

After a prisoner completed his or her trials, the emperor granted a pardon, and prison administrators released the free man or woman on the northeastern border of China. Every year, additional death row inmates joined the experiments. Each area of experimentation involved many years of trial and many thousands of prisoners. Some prisoners participated in studies of ingredients that were not effective, and their test treatments did not cure them. Lord Liu ordered that the experiments should return these patients to health when they had identified the most effective cure for their illness. Subsequently, the emperor granted the prisoners pardon, and the administrators released them.

Summary of Lord Liu Chun's Research

Subject of Research	Participants per Trial*	Duration of Research**
1. Cancer	200	More than 30 years
2. Diabetes	200	More than 13 years
3. Lethargy and physical weakness	200	Several years
4. Energy in the stomach (hunger)	200 older males	Several years
5. Influenza	200	5 years

6. Erectile dysfunction	200 males	5 years
7. Hepatitis	200	4–5 years
8. Cholera	200	5–6 years
9. Bruise and injuries	200	14 years
10. Epilepsy, schizophrenia, drug addiction	200	Several years
11. Chronic enteritis, gastric ulcer	200	Several years
12. Aplastic anemia, endometrorrhagia	200	Several years
13. Preventative food therapy	200	Several years
14. Nephritis, cardiomyopathy	200	More than 30 years
15. Acne, appendicitis	200	Several years
16. Arteriosclerosis, coronary heart disease, apoplexy, stroke	200	Several years
17. Ten points to enhancement of life	200	13 years
18. Rheumatoid arthritis, lupus, hysteromyoma	200	14 years
19. Bronchitis	200	Several years
20. Pregnancy	30 males and 30 females	Unknown
21. Problems with alcohol	30	Unknown
22. Advantages of meat soup and the disadvantage of eating meat	180	Unknown
23. Study of human yin and yang energy	40	14 years
24. Methods of pain relief	Not described	Unknown
25. (a) Study of chemical calcium tablets	30 older males	Unknown

(b) Negative side effects of chemical calcium tablets	37	25 years
26. Treatment of patients with multiple diseases	20	Unknown
27. Aphrodisiac drugs and early death	70 (60+ years of age)	Unknown
28. Water intake	Not known	More than 3 years
29. Study of 5,611 herbs		
(a) Research on drugs	336,660 (5,611 herbs for study × 20 people per trial × minimum of 3 trials per herb)	More than 60 years (Lord Liu assigned fifty medical doctors specifically to this project.)
(b) Drug therapeutic effect	4,568 herbs × 20 (number of trials not known)	25 years
30. Study of acu-points and acu-meridians	100	66 years (Lord Liu assigned 7 medical doctors specifically to this project.)

* Unless otherwise noted, participant groups included both male and female subjects.
** Length of time that a remedy was researched. During this period, researchers performed many trials.

During research in 1410, Lord Liu Chun discovered that many of the medicines he tested appeared in medical journals but had not been subjected to any form of scientific testing. He spent more than sixty-six years researching each of the 5,611 herbs, minerals, and animal products known in traditional Chinese medicine. He subjected each item to vigorous testing and many trials were performed to find the effectiveness of each remedy.

Researchers gathered twenty people in a group to perform a series of four experiments:

1. They mixed a specific herb with congee (porridge) made from millet (第一步，把药材粉末拌入小米粥里让犯人吃).

2. They ground the herb into a powder and mixed in the patient's bathwater (第二步，把药材粉末放在水里让犯人浸泡).

3. They burnt the herb and instructed the patient to inhale the fumes (第三步，把药材粉末燃烧让犯人呼吸).

4. The patient ingested the herb with hunger-inducing soup (第四步，把药材粉末与北山楂，广木香共煮让犯人喝).

By testing these different applications, Lord Liu Chun identified the most efficient methods to cure illness. For example, to cure fever, Lord Liu and his researchers selected an herb that would lower body temperature. They administered this herb until the patient felt cold. Then they tested other herbs to identify the herb that would raise the body temperature. In this way, they found the most efficient herbs for cooling and heating.

Another test researched the best method for retaining body fluid and nourishing the yin energy.[ii] Researchers tested many herbal remedies, including: *Radix Glehniae* (沙参sha shen); *Herba Dendrobii* (石斛shi hu); *Radix Paeoniae Alba* (白芍bai shao); *Rhizoma Polygonati* (黄精huang jing); *Rhizoma Polygonati Odorati* (玉竹yu zhu); *Radix Asparagi* (天冬tian dong); *Radix Ophiopogonis* (麦冬mai dong); *Fructus Ligustri Lucidi* (女真子nu zhen zi); *Plastrum Testudinis* (龟板gui ban); *Carapax Trionycis* (鳖甲bie jia); *Bulbus*

---

ii The "contrary treatment," one of the basic therapeutic principles in Traditional Chinese Medicine (TCM) was developed in the light of the opposition between yin and yang. For example, the treatment of cold disease with drugs hot in nature means to use heat (yang) to control cold (yin), while the treatment of febrile disease with drugs cold in nature means to use drugs (yin) to restrict heat (Yang).

Lilli (百合bai he); and *Radix Panacis Quinquefolii* (西洋参Xi yang shen). After many experiments, Lord Liu concluded that pork skin soup was the most effective approach to maintaining body fluid and nourishing the yin energy.

In this way, by trial and error, Lord Liu and his researchers identified the best medicines for various ailments.

Lord Liu Chun commented, "Many people think that this research is cumbersome and a waste of time (是药皆试，或以为愚，非也，莫以流言为是，必欲亲知). These trials must be done because the properties of each ingredient must be known. Performing this research makes me very tired and pressured, however, I will persist until completion (以囚试药力者，其浩繁非比，余衰于此矣)."

Despite the medieval concepts of feudalism, morality, and corporal punishment prevailing in his time, Lord Liu Chun requested the return to good health and release of the prisoners upon their completion of the experiments. Although his requests resulted in freedom for hundreds of thousands of people, hundreds of death row inmates also died in the experimentation process. We do not wish to debate the morality of a process that took place in a feudal dynasty six hundred years ago. We would only like to pay a sincere tribute to those who died and hope that some scientists today might use this data to search for cures for mankind, thus ensuring that they did not lose their lives in vain.

Chapter 3
Hunger: The Key to Curing Illness

Energy in the Stomach (Hunger) (胃气)

In many developed countries, the discussion of hunger is often associated with eating disorders related to physical and emotional issues (including obesity, anorexia, and bulimia). Mental health professionals encourage us to distinguish between emotional hunger and physical hunger.

In 1992, Montana's Department of Public Health and Human Services sponsored the Eat Right Montana coalition to urge citizens to listen to their hunger cues and use their natural ability to regulate food intake signals of hunger and satiety.[1] Some people believe that intuitive eating—learning to listen to and eat according to those signals—creates a healthy relationship between food, mind, and body.

Thousands of years ago, as ancient Chinese civilization flourished, simple characters evolved from pictographs, and compound characters were formed to accommodate the increase in complex thought and expression. Somehow, the early Chinese had an insight to the true meaning and importance of hunger. The Chinese character for hunger (饿) is a compound of two basic characters: eat (食) and me (我). If a body is experiencing true hunger and has no extraneous source of fuel, it will tap into its own stored reserves for energy. In essence, it will eat itself. Traditional Chinese doctors propose that, if one has *energy in the stomach*, one will survive, but when there is no *energy in the stomach*, no cure will be effective (有胃气则生，无胃气则死).

Energy in the stomach refers to the state of physical hunger or appetite, without signs of indigestion such as bloating, nausea, or diarrhea. If one has hunger, the digestive system is strong, and the body can absorb nutrients. If metabolism is strong, the body can combat disease and sickness. Without hunger, the metabolism is not active and the body cannot absorb nutrients or self-regulate to combat disease.

Many people confuse appetite with hunger. One may wish to eat, but it may be a craving, which is a form of emotional hunger. True hunger, a good digestive system, and a high metabolism allow food consumption without weight gain.

There are two categories of hunger: emotional hunger and physical hunger. Emotional hunger is sudden and urgent. It occurs automatically with cravings for a specific kind of food and can be dictated by one's mood. It is essentially an "above the neck" sensation, and the person may feel remorse after eating. Physical hunger has a more gradual onset and is more constant. The feeling originates from the stomach, and there is no desire for a specific food. After eating, one notices the feeling of fullness. When responding to physical hunger, one is in control and can make logical decisions when eating.

In Okinawa, Japan, well known for the Okinawa diet and the relative longevity of its people, "*Hara Hachi Bu*" is a well-known adage. It means, "Stomach eighty percent full."[2] The Chinese suggest eating until one is 70 percent full. According to the Western concept of "intuitive hunger," one eats until the feeling of hunger is gone.[3]

In general, developed countries do not experience famine. Food is plentiful and enjoyed too much. True hunger is almost nonexistent; rather, obesity is a prominent concern. Studies have shown that mice receiving fewer calories or who are subjected to intermittent fasting live longer with less chance of disease.

Lord Liu Chun once said that *hunger is the key* to curing illness. When treating a patient, the first step is to stimulate hunger. This creates good energy in the stomach and good digestion to optimize absorption. Without true hunger, the body will not efficiently absorb medication. Lord Liu Chun believed that, if one did not feel hunger, there would be no chance for his or her disease to be cured (人无胃气不治).

Lord Liu and his colleagues discussed in depth the initial symptoms of illness. The first symptom is the loss of hunger. They observed that many patients with cancer and cardiovascular problems experienced no hunger for several months prior to the diagnosis.

The following chart, taken from the article, "Tumor-Induced Effects on Nutritional Status," published by the National Cancer Institute, documents recent efforts to identify a drug that would effectively induce increased appetite in tumor patients. The information from the chart indicates that Western researchers recognize the importance of appetite in tumor patients, although so far they have identified no effective medication.

Commonly Prescribed Medications

Drug Category	Common Drug Used	Comments
Progestational agents	megestrol acetate medroxyprogesterone	Multiple investigations report appetite stimulant activity and weight gain with use. Body composition of weight gain indicates *increased body fat stores instead of lean body tissue. Increased risk of thromboembolism* with doses >800 mg/day is an apparent trend. Studies suggest improved effectiveness in patients with better digestive function; therefore, targeted nutritional strategies such as digestive enzymes or elemental diets may be useful.
Glucocorticoids	Dexamethasone Methylprednisolone Prednisolone	Mechanism of appetite stimulation is unknown but likely related to anti-inflammatory and euphoric actions. Studies report positive but *short-lived effects* on clinical outcomes such as appetite and quality of life, with minimal or no effect on weight gain. Risk of adverse effects such as muscle wasting and immunosuppressant limit use for long-term use for appetite stimulation.
Cannabinoids	Dronabinol	*Inconsistent evidence* of clinical effectiveness in cancer patients. Studies of dronabinol alone or with megestrol acetate have not shown superior benefit in promoting weight gain and appetite.

Drug Category	Common Drug Used	Comments
Antihistamines	Cyproheptadine	*Not studied well* in cancer patients. A randomized placebo-controlled trial in patients with advanced cancer reported no difference in weight changes and progressive weight loss in both groups. Sedation is a frequent adverse effect that may limit usefulness in cancer patients.
Antidepressants/ antipsychotics	Mirtazapine Olanzapine	Clinical data supporting routine use in cancer patients are lacking. *Further studies are needed.*
Anti-inflammatory agents	Thalidomide Pentoxifylline Melatonin omega-3 fatty acids (EPA)	All have been shown to decrease tumor necrosis factor α (TNFα). Mixed results in clinical trials regarding weight gain and appetite stimulation. One published randomized placebo-controlled trial evaluated the safety and efficacy of thalidomide, 200 mg daily, in patients with advanced pancreatic cancer and weight loss of at least 10% of premorbid weight. Thalidomide group showed a significant difference in weight loss compared with the placebo group, indicating the drug's ability to safely decrease weight loss and loss of lean body mass in the patients studied. Preliminary clinical studies and laboratory studies of the polyunsaturated fatty acid eicosapentaenoic acid (EPA) have suggested a benefit to cancer patients; however, *subsequent large comparative studies failed to reproduce this benefit.*
Metabolic inhibitors	hydrazine sulfate	*Not approved by the U.S. Food and Drug Administration (FDA)* for marketing in the United States.

Drug Category	Common Drug Used	Comments
Anabolic agents	Oxandrolone	Used in an attempt to stimulate muscle anabolism. *Limited published reports* of successful appetite stimulation in cancer patients.
	nandrolone decanoate	
	Fluoxymesterone	

Reprinted with permission from the National Cancer Institute, "Tumor-Induced Effects on Nutritional Status, April 10, 2008, http://www.cancer.gov/cancertopics/pdq/supportivecare/nutrition/HealthProfessional/page3; italics added.

It's clear from the comments on this chart that modern medicine still needs to identify a highly effective appetite-induction drug.

To develop a technique to induce hunger and rekindle appetite, Lord Liu Chun conducted years of tests of different herbs on death row prisoners. His appetite-inducing soup, containing shan zha (Hawthorn山楂) and guang mu xiang (*Costus* root) (广木香), is the product of his trials.

Lord Liu Chun's descendent, Dr. Liu Hong Zhang, has recreated the experiments using dogs as test subjects. His experiments prove that the appetite-inducing soup is more effective than most Eastern and Western drugs.

When a patient has regained his hunger, the best food to consume is soup of freshwater fish or minced beef. These soups must be simmered for twelve hours to extract the soluble protein. On a daily basis, Dr. Liu also prescribes one liter of fresh fruit juice and a diet high in fiber to aid in detoxification.

The practice of fasting is common in many cultures and religions. Muslims fast every year for one month during their observation of Ramadan. Fervent Buddhist monks do not eat solid food after the noon hour.[4] Christians also practice fasting during Lent and at other dates of religious observance. Many religions discourage excess in materialistic possession as well as in dietary consumption. Perhaps the early fathers of these religions recognized the spiritual and physical benefits of moderation.

According to Dr. Shanti B. Rangwani, who touts the therapeutic benefits of fasting the golden rule of dietetics states, "To keep healthy one must always keep a little hunger."[5]

Lord Liu Chun's theories are still innovative by today's standards. To prevent disease, one needs to be hungry. Modern science has documented this important aspect of treatment. Nevertheless, modern health care practitioners still generally ignore it. Lord Liu Chun has proposed four ways to create hunger:

1. Drink one liter of cold water every morning upon waking.
2. At dinnertime, consume only meat soup and fruit juice.
3. Practice abdominal and neck-stretching exercises to prevent osteoporosis in the vertebrae, which would hinder blood circulation to the hypothalamus.
4. Drink appetite-inducing soup if the appetite is weak.

In Chinese medicine, there are traditionally recognized physical symptoms of the loss of hunger. Lord Liu identified the following physical symptoms as further evidence of this condition:

1. The patient's tongue is covered by a thick, white film, and the texture is comparable to cooked chicken meat.
2. The scrotum of a male patient is flaccid (阴囊绵软无纹), and the vagina of a female patient is poorly lubricated (阴户干涩如纸).
3. Any inflammation on the skin shows no signs of pus (黄脓).
4. The patient walks by concentrating all his or her body weight on the heels. This indicates that the spine is very stiff and the patient has very poor circulation, especially in the region of the neck vertebrae.

Appetite-Inducing Soup

For thousands of years, traditional Chinese doctors have believed that, if one's stomach has energy, one will feel hungry and life will be sustained. The existence of hunger is considered to be an indicator of good metabolism and the body's ability to absorb. If the body can absorb nutrients from food, it will also be able to absorb medicine, and the right medicines will be able to prevent illness.

According to Lord Liu Chun, a patient without hunger will not benefit from taking medicine. Inducing hunger, therefore, is the crucial first step in preventing illness and recovery. (Recent discoveries of hormones affecting hunger,such as leptin, orexins ,ghrelin and obestatin shine additional light on Lord Liu Chun's concept of hunger.)

After Lord Liu Chun proved this theory with detailed research, Imperial Physicians adopted this approach.

Test 1: Finding the Right Ingredients

In 1409, Lord Liu Chun began his experiments on energy in the stomach. Researchers gave two hundred elderly prisoners dosages of limestone water in the morning, afternoon, and evening.

They designed a diet consisting of only rice and vegetables (no animal protein) to cause malnutrition. After one month, all the prisoners had lost their appetite and desire to eat. These prisoners were then divided into twenty groups of ten to test the concoctions listed below in an effort to induce hunger.

Concoctions Tested in Effort to Find Hunger-inducing Herbs

Group	Decoction	Latin Name	Chinese Name
1	gou qi	*Fructus Lycii*	枸杞汤
2	ma huang	*Herba Ephedrae*	麻黄汤
3	xiao hui xiang	*Fructus Foeniculi*	小茴香汤

4	ren shen	*Radix Ginseng*	人参汤
5	jin yin hua	*Flos Lonicerae*	金银花汤
6	zhi shi	*Fructus Auranti Immaturus*	枳实汤
7	ci shi	*Magnetitum*	磁石汤
8	sha shen	*Radix Glehniae*	沙参汤
9	wu mei	*Fructus Mume*	乌梅汤
10	di yu	*Radix Sanguisorbae*	地榆汤
11	dang gui	*Radix Angelicae Sinensis*	当归汤
12	zhu ling	*Polyporus Umbellatus*	猪苓汤
13	jing jie	*Herba Schizonepetae*	荆芥汤
14	qing huo	*Rhizoma Seu Radix Notopterygii*	羌活汤
15	chuan bei mu	*Bulbus Fritillariae Cirrhosae*	川贝母汤
16	mu li	*Concha Ostreae*	牡蛎汤
17	cao jue ming	*Cassia Tora L*	草决明汤
18	chuan xiong	*Rhizoma Ligustici*	川芎汤
19	bei shan zha	*Fructus Crataegi* (Haw-thorn)	山楂汤
20	shi jun zi	*Fructus Quisqualis*	使君子汤

In the studies, Groups 6 and 19 began to regain their appetite.

After these experiments, researchers tested other herbs on the same groups.

Test 2: Finding the Right Ingredients

Concoctions Tested in Effort to Find Hunger-inducing Herbs

Group	Decoction	Latin Name	Chinese Name
1	guang mu xiang	*Costus* root	广木香汤
2	yun mu xiang	Common *Aucklandia*	云木香汤
3	chuan mu xiang	*Sichuan Dolomiaea* root	川木香汤
4	qing mu xiang	*Radix Aristolochiae*	青木香汤
5	xiang fu	*Rhizoma Cyperi*	香附汤
6	wu yao	*Radix Linderae*	乌药汤
7	chen xiang	*Lignum Aquilariae Resi-natum*	沉香汤

8	zhi shi	*Fructus Aurantii Immaturus*	枳实汤
9	hou po	*Contex Mangoliae Officinalis*	厚朴汤
10	fo shou	*Fructus Citri Sarcodactylis*	佛手汤
11	sheng bei shan zha guo	Raw *Fructus Crataegi*	生北山楂果汤
12	sheng bei shan zha tang	Sliced Raw *Fructus Crataegi*	生北山楂片汤
13	chao bei shan zha pian	Fried *Fructus Crataegi*	炒北山楂片汤
14	sheng nan shan zha guo	*Fructus Crataegi* (from Southern China)	生南山楂果汤
15	mai ya	*Fructus Hordei Germinatus*	麦芽汤
16	gu ya	*Fructus Setariae Germinatus*	谷芽汤
17	shen you	N/A	神粬汤
18	ji nei jin	*Endothelium Corneum Gigeriae Galli*	鸡内金汤
19	ya nei jin	N/A	鸭内金汤
20	lai fu zi	*Semen Raphani*	莱菔子汤

In this study, patients in Groups 1 and 11 regained their hunger before the other groups. Further studies revealed that the herbs researchers used in tests 1.19 and 2.1, *shan zha* (Hawthorn) and *guang mu xiang* (*Costus* root), were the most effective.

Test 3: Finding the Correct Dosage

Now that the researchers had found the right concoctions, they had to determine what quantities would work best to induce their patients' hunger.

Dosages of Hunger-inducing Herbs Tested

Group	Bei shan zha (*Fructus Crataegi/* Hawthorn 北山楂) (Dosage in taels*)	guang mu xiang (*Costus* Root 广木香) (Dosage in taels*)
1	1	1
2	2	1

3	3	1
4	4	1
5	5	1
6	1	2
7	2	2
8	3	2
9	4	2
10	5	2
11	1	3
12	2	3
13	3	3
14	4	3
15	5	3
16	1	4
17	2	4
18	3	4
19	4	4
20	5	4

*1 tael = 31.25 grams

Researchers then used patients in groups 1 through 20 to find the correct amount of bei shan zha and guang mu xiang to be administered. Four taels of bei shan zha and two taels of guang mu xiang were found to be the correct dosage. The experiments were conducted repeatedly for verification.

Test 4: Modern Testing

Dr. Liu Hong Zhang (刘弘章), a physician trained in Western medicine and a twenty-fourth generation descendent of Lord Liu, has recreated this experiment using dogs as patients.

Zhang placed two electrodes on the dogs' hypothalamuses to monitor brain activity and planted a tube in the dogs' stomach to monitor stomach secretion.

1. Zhang gave the dogs enzymes. He detected no abnormal activity in the hypothalamus or the rest of the brain. The dogs' stomachs produced digestive liquids. Zhang

concluded that the enzymes only assisted in the digestive process; they did not create hunger.

2. Zhang gave steroids to the dogs to increase their metabolism. The dogs' hypothalamuses, brains, and stomachs showed no change. Initially, the dogs exhibited some increase in appetite, but when they were satiated with steroids, they lost all desire to eat.

3. Zhang gave the dogs ginseng, coffee, and tea. Their hypothalamuses and stomachs showed no abnormal activity. The brain, however, seemed very stimulated and excited. The dogs were nervous and did not want to eat.

4. Zhang gave the dogs the appetite-inducing soup. Their hypothalamuses showed an increased volume of electricity. Their stomachs produced significant digestive liquids and their brain waves remained constant. The dogs began to eat and never seemed to be full.

5. The dogs were given only bei shan zha (Hawthorn). Their hypothalamuses showed no change, their stomachs secreted little digestive liquid, and their brainwaves remained constant. The dogs only ate small quantities. Zhang concluded that using bei shan zha as the sole ingredient was not enough.

6. Next, Zhang tested guang mu xiang. The dogs' hypothalamuses showed great volumes of electricity, their production of digestive liquids did not increase much, and their brain waves remained constant. The dogs only had appetite for soft foods; they did not want bones or food that required chewing.

This research indicated that stimulating the hypothalamus and creating appetite or stomach energy requires a combination of bei shan zha and guang mu xiang. Western researchers have also studied the hunger-regulating properties of the hypothalamus.

According to HerbMed, an electric database of herbs that compiles data about scientific research on the use of herbs to promote health, researchers have thoroughly studied bei shan zha (Hawthorn) in thirty-two clinical trials, twenty-four animal experiments, and fifty-six analytical chemistry tests.[6] Guang mu xiang (*Costus* root) is also well known in ancient medicinal practices, being a primary ingredient in Indian Siddha medicine. It is used to treat ailments of eyes, stomach, neck, jaws, tongue, and mouth and also can be used to treat fever, edema, wheezing, hemorrhoids, and spermaturia.[7]

Preparing Appetite-Inducing Soup

After soaking the herbs, simmer them at low heat in a glass, heatproof pot. You can consume the soup warm or at room temperature.

Ingredients

100 grams bei shan zha

50 grams guang mu xiang

1 liter fresh water

10 dried red dates (optional)

Directions

(1) Place the dry ingredients in a heatproof, glass pot. Cover with cold water and soak for thirty minutes.

(2) Drain and cover with 1 liter of fresh water. Bring to boil then reduce heat.

(3) Simmer for thirty minutes and strain into a glass container.

(4) Add 1 liter of cold water to the herbs and reboil. Simmer for thirty minutes.

(5) Strain into the glass container.

This should produce around 1.5 liters of soup. Drink it in one hundred-milliliter portions warmed or at room temperature, preferably finishing the soup within one day. Discard any remaining soup. Do not add sweetener, sugar, or honey. To improve the taste, you may add ten dried red dates during the cooking process.

For children under the age of fourteen, adults weighing less than 110 pounds, or patients over the age of seventy, reduce the dosage by half.

Cancer patients whose appetites are returning should continue drinking the soup at least every other day.

Once the appetite has stabilized, discourage overeating. In the evening, consume only meat soup or fruit juices. Feeling hungry is an important step in the body's return to good health.

Translating Chinese Medicine for Western Cultures

In 1953, Russian experts called a meeting at the Ministry of Health in China. They invited well-known traditional Chinese doctors, including Dr. Liu Shi Kui, a descendent of Lord Liu Chun.

During the meeting, these experts asked how the appetite-inducing soup could elevate an individual's hunger. Dr. Liu replied that bei shan zha and guang mu xiang could rekindle appetite. The Russian experts argued that protein enzymes could have the same effect and questioned the need for bei shan zha and guang mu xiang.

They asked why bovine flexor tendon could inhibit cancer from spreading. Dr. Liu answered that the gelatin of the tendon soup could enclose the cancer cells and inhibit further growth. The Russian experts laughed and suggested the use of glue instead of the tendon.

They questioned the effectiveness of the Liu family cancer remedy, kong yan san (控岩散) in curing cancer. Dr. Liu answered that cancer is a symptom of excessive heat in blood and rampant growth of blood vessels (angiogenesis, 血热妄行). Shark's gallbladder is the main ingredient of kong yan san, which reduces the heat in the blood.

Again the Russians questioned the validity of this method and commented that the Chinese doctor did not know what he was doing or why.

At that time, Dr. Liu Shi Kui knew how to prevent cancer using Chinese medical methods, but he could not explain the methodology in Western medical terms. In the last decade, the translation of Chinese herbs, medical processes, and cultural traditions into Western terms has become possible through improved linguistic and cultural exchange. *Lord Liu Chun's Secrets of Longevity* presents Lord Liu Chun's methodologies in a new, non-Chinese format for the first time.

Chapter 4
Lord Liu's Ten Steps to the Enhancement of Life

Lord Liu Chun's Research

After being usurped by his own uncle, the second Ming emperor, Zhu Yun Wen (明朝皇帝朱允文), retired to lead a long and simple life, dying peacefully in 1471, at the age of ninety-four. Lord Liu took notice of this remarkable lifespan. After studying the second Ming emperor's life, Lord Liu made six observations about the emperor's lifestyle.

The Emperor, unlike many of his predecessors:

1. Did not take any elixirs prepared by the Taoist priests
2. Ate simple foods
3. Led a very active life, performing daily activities and chores without any help from staff
4. Became a monk in his later years, consequently detaching himself from his family and leading an ascetic life
5. Showed contentment and did not harbor any hatred or desire for revenge, even against the uncle who overthrew him on the throne
6. Enjoyed art and nature, expressing himself in poetry

The second Ming emperor inspired Lord Liu in his quest for a healthy lifestyle. Lord Liu began his research by inducing the symptoms of deficiency in yin and vital essence (阴精亏虚，胃气不足), creating patients who lacked vitality and appetite. He divided two hundred death row inmates into two groups of a hundred people each and used them for the study.

Group A

Members of the first group consumed the following diet to deteriorate the body:

1. Limewater (石灰水) (Researchers intended to cause inflammation of the digestive tract and indigestion (制造胃肠损伤).
2. Meatless diet of vegetables and rice (Researchers prescribed this diet to reduce protein and cause malnutrition.)

Lord Liu and his team further divided the first group into ten groups of ten. They gave each group additional food items and instructed them to adhere to a specific constraint. They assigned the final group an accumulation of all the previous conditions and the additional challenge of psychological abuse to weaken their mental health.

1. Researchers gave the first group tea made from one catty (about one and a quarter pounds) of tea leaves.
2. They gave the second group tea made from one catty of tea leaves and one catty of sugar.
3. The third group drank tea with sugar, plus one catty of strong distilled liquor.
4. The fourth group drank tea with sugar and liquor and ate as chili peppers in their rice, as well.

5. The fifth group drank with sugar and liquor and ate chili peppers in their rice. Researchers did not allow them to nap in the afternoon.

6. The sixth group drank tea with sugar and liquor. In addition to chili peppers in their rice, they ate half a catty of pork fat. Researchers didn't allow this group to nap in the afternoon either.

7. The seventh group drank tea with sugar and liquor. They ate chili peppers in their rice and pork fat. In addition to the napping restriction, this group could not walk or exercise. Researchers instructed them to sit cross-legged all day.

8. The eighth group drank tea with sugar and liquor and ate chili peppers in their rice and pork fat. Researchers didn't allow them to nap, walk, or exercise. The group consumed additional toxic Taoist elixirs in the evening.

9. The ninth group drank tea with sugar and liquor, ate chili peppers in their rice and pork fat, and consumed toxic Taoist elixirs in the evening. Researchers did not allow this group to nap, walk, or exercise. In addition, they instructed the group to have frequent sexual intercourse with female inmates.

10. The tenth group drank tea with sugar and liquor, ate chili peppers in their rice and pork fat, and consumed toxic Taoist elixirs in the evening. This group could not nap, walk, or exercise. Researchers instructed them to have frequent sexual intercourse, and the soldiers subjected them to psychological abuse. Soldiers insulted the inmates to weaken their minds and self-esteem (每天喝一斤，再加一斤糖，一斤蒸馏酒，饭菜之中加辣椒；中午不许睡眠；临睡觉吃半斤猪肥膘；白天盘腿而坐，晚上吃炼丹；每天夜里给一个女犯人去性交。).

Summary of Experiments with Subjects with Induced Deficiency in Yin and Yang Essence: Groups A and B

Group A	1	2	3	4	5	6	7	8	9	10
Tea made from $1\frac{1}{4}$ pounds of tea leaves	√	√	√	√	√	√	√	√	√	√
$1\frac{1}{4}$ pounds sugar		√	√	√	√	√	√	√	√	√
$1\frac{1}{4}$ pounds (approximately 500 cc) distilled liquor			√	√	√	√	√	√	√	√
Chili peppers in rice				√	√	√	√	√	√	√
No afternoon nap					√	√	√	√	√	√
¾ pound of fatty pork						√	√	√	√	√
No exercise							√	√	√	√
Taoist elixirs								√	√	√
Daily intercourse									√	√
Psychological abuse										√

Group B

Researchers also prescribed the hundred members of the second group a special diet of two items:

1. Appetite-inducing soup
2. Beef soup

In addition, researchers divided this group into ten groups of ten. They assigned the individual groups in Group B the same conditions as the corresponding ten groups in Group A.

Conclusions from Research

After a month, the members of Group A exhibited signs of rapid aging. They were exhausted, and their health was deteriorating. Group B exhibited similar, yet less severe results.

After repeating this experiment in several trials, Lord Liu was able to draw specific conclusions about aging from each of the conditions of the ten groups. He observed that people age faster from:

1. Malnutrition
2. Diuretics (from drinking great amounts of tea, 利尿)
3. Yin deficiency (from excessive consumption of sugar, 阴虚)
4. Liver and stomach problems (from a high level of alcohol intake)
5. Excessive heat energy in blood circulation (from consuming hot foods like chili, 血热)
6. Lack of rest
7. Indigestion (from the consumption of fatty foods)
8. Lack of exercise
9. Consumption of toxins (from the Taoist elixirs)
10. Negative emotional state (caused by psychological abuse)

From his experiments Lord Liu concluded that in order to lead a long and healthy life, *one must live an orderly life.* Simply relying on medicine is not sufficient; being healthy requires adopting a healthy lifestyle.

Ten Points to the Enhancement of Life

For many generations, members of the Liu family have followed their ancestor's philosophy and have enjoyed very long and healthy lives. Lord Liu formulated a ten-point strategy crucial to the maintenance of a healthy lifestyle:

1. Perform morning exercises upon waking and while still in bed. Following a set of eighteen prescribed exercises, consume one liter of cold water every morning. According to Lord Liu, energy level in the stomach is lowest in the morning, and drinking cold water will stimulate hunger. The cold water also aids in the cleansing of the digestive tract by stimulating intestinal movement. Start with a smaller amount of cold water and gradually increase the amount up to one liter. Children and menstruating women can consume smaller quantities.

2. The heaviest meal of the day should be the midday meal—lunch. It should consist of a diet high in protein, vegetable, and fiber. Avoid solid meat; instead, consume liquefied protein in the form of meat soup (tendon, meat, fish, or skin). Lord Liu also recommended foods containing fiber such as corn, yam, barley, and beans. Avoid white and glutinous rice.

3. Take a thirty-minute walk after eating the midday meal. Follow the walk with a nap.

4. Consume fresh fruit juices after the nap to replenish the vitamins in the body. Consume about one liter of juice throughout the day.

5. Perform vigorous exercise in the late afternoon. The exercise must induce perspiration and include loud vocalizations (Kiai喊叫). Lord Liu Chun believed that simply performing qi gong was insufficient; he recommended muscle-strengthening exercises such as weight lifting.

6. Do not eat solid foods during the rest of the day. *Consume only meat soup and fruit juices (or fruits) during the*

evening meal. Lord Liu was a devout Buddhist, and he arrived at this conclusion after many years of Buddhist practice. Buddhists believed that one should eat to live and not live to eat.

7. Soak feet in warm water before bedtime. The warm water stimulates acupressure points, resulting in a restful sleep.

8. Practice spirituality (宗教信仰), as it is vital to mental equilibrium.

9. Men should ejaculate only once a month (精气足而长寿, 房事每月一次), so as to optimize the vivacity of the sperm and produce the best offspring.

10. Irrigate the colon once a month to rid the body of toxins.

Liu Chun and Western Research

The ten conclusions that Lord Liu Chun made about the enhancement of life do not exist collectively in the world of Western medicine, although individual aspects have been subjected to medical discussion and analysis. The aspects that both Lord Liu Chun and Western scientists have explored are described below.

Morning Routine: Exercise and Water

1. Morning exercises in bed (养生之松骨运动18式):

    From observations of the emperor's soldiers, Lord Liu Chun found that, when the soldiers awoke after six or more hours of nighttime sleep, their bodies were at least a half inch longer than they were when they had gone to bed. Such was not the case with people who slept less than six hours. The concept was that, at nighttime, people tend to be shorter because their joints have born pressure during the day. After six hours of sleep, the joints and tendons relax and return to normal.

Lord Liu Chun also determined that a person who performed exercises in bed upon waking would be able to stretch the tendons more efficiently, maintain better joint lubrication (骨囊液体), and improve circulation.

In our modern world, few scientists have attempted to study whether there is an optimal time for exercise. Six hundred years ago, Lord Liu Chun found that, upon waking in the morning, before rising and subjecting one's body to the compression caused by the Earth's gravity, the body is in the best condition to benefit from particular exercises. One exercise he proposed is a neck stretch that requires a pillow. In the prone position, gravity does not compress the spine. One can practice low-impact exercises and minimize any harm to the body. Once a person stands up or sits, gravity and body weigh affect the condition in which he or she exercises. Lord Liu Chun used a skeleton to demonstrate this.

From his research, he created an exercise of eighteen movements. We will discuss these exercises further in another publication.

2. Water intake:

Water is one of the essential sources of life; without it, any living creature is susceptible to disease and even to death. The amount of water that people should consume is often disputed.

Lord Liu Chun performed many studies to identify the ideal volume of water that human beings require. He divided a group of two hundred prison inmates into five groups of forty people each and assigned each group a different amount of water to consume daily. He gave the first group one liter. Each subsequent drank an additional liter.

Within three years, the first and second groups succumbed to many diseases. Over the same time period, the people who drank three liters of water were occasionally diagnosed with diseases (日饮3升水者，不越三年，偶发疾病；日饮4升水者，越三年矣，不发病也). Members of the fourth and fifth groups did not suffer from any disease. From that point on, the Ming dynasty supplied its soldiers with at least four liters of water daily.

Lord Liu Chun revised his treatment for the other patients in the following manner:

- One liter of cold water in the morning
- One bowl of meat soup for breakfast
- Water or soy bean soup at 10:00 AM
- One bowl of meat soup for lunch
- One half liter of water or soybean soup following the afternoon nap
- Fresh fruit juice after 4:00 PM
- Fresh fruit juice or meat soup at 6:00 PM
- Cold water at 8:00 PM

The total daily intake of liquid should be more than four liters.

In modern times, researchers from the University of Iowa have also concluded that a person should consume at least four liters of liquid every day. Alcohol, tea, and coffee should not be included in this minimum because they are diuretics and result in the depletion of liquids.[1]

Eating: Light Meals, High Fiber, and Cooking Methods

1. Hunger and eating a light dinner:

   In 2005, the Laboratories of Cardiovascular Sciences and of Neurosciences of the National Institute on Aging, through the Intramural Research Program at the National Institutes of Health in Baltimore, Maryland, conducted research on heart failure titled "Cardioprotection by Intermittent Fasting in Rats." The research concluded that, "IF [intermittent fasting] protects the heart from ischemic injury and attenuates post-MI cardiac remodeling, likely via antiapoptotic and anti-inflammatory mechanisms."[2]

   In 2006, the National Institute on Aging published a research paper on caloric restriction and intermittent fasting. The experimentation suggests that patterns of food consumption affect heart rate and blood pressure in rats. The research also indicates that the "additional cardiovascular benefit of DR [dietary restriction] merits further studies of this potential effect in humans."[3]

   Strict Buddhists adhere to the belief that the purpose of food is to provide sustenance and not pleasure. Traditionally, the last meal of the day for Buddhist monks and nuns is the midday meal. They refrain from eating solid foods from afternoon until the following dawn. Buddha famously said, "Wisely reflecting we use this almsfood, not for fun, not for pleasure, not for fattening and not for beautification. But only for the maintenance and nourishment of this body, for keeping it healthy, for helping with the holy life, thinking this: I will allay hunger without overeating, so that I may continue to live blamelessly and at ease."

2. High fiber intake:

Fiber can be classified into two categories: soluble and insoluble. Soluble fiber aids in lowering cholesterol and controlling blood sugar in diabetics. This type of fiber can be found in legumes; oat bran; oatmeal; flax; barley; and pectin-rich fruits, like apples, strawberries, and citrus. Insoluble fiber, or roughage, has been known to aid in lowering the occurrence of certain cancers, preventing constipation, and improving other bowel conditions. This type of fiber includes wheat bran; whole wheat products; brown rice; fruit peel; and vegetables, including carrots, broccoli, and peas.

In 2007, the University of Leeds completed a study that concluded that "fiber ... lowers breast cancer risk." The case study included 35,000 women; one group ate thirty grams of fiber each day, while the other ate less than twenty grams. The results of the research revealed that the group who ate twenty grams or less of fiber each day had twice the risk of breast cancer compared with those who ate thirty grams daily. A thirty-gram portion of fiber represents a serving of high-fiber cereal, a whole-grain snack, and five servings of fruits or vegetables daily. After menopause, however, the results vary.[4]

In 2003, the *Canadian Journal of Dietetic Practice and Research* published research on the effects of soluble fiber on cholesterol. Men and women with moderate levels of blood cholesterol were subject to two different diets: a low-fat diet, where fat comprised less than 30 percent of the daily caloric intake, and a high-soluble fiber diet, where subjects added ten grams of soluble fiber to their diet. Researchers compared the effects of both diets and found that both produced a similar effect of successfully lowering the blood cholesterol levels.[5]

In 2002, the *Journal of Small Animal Practice* published research the University of Glasgow performed on the "influence of a high fiber diet on glycaemic control and quality of life in dogs with diabetes mellitus." The researchers found that a diet high in fiber could aid in glycemic control and improve the life of dogs with diabetes mellitus.[6]

3. Cooking methods:

In 2007, the Mount Sinai School of Medicine published research that advised, "Keeping the heat down and *maintaining the water content in food reduces AGE levels ... particularly steaming, boiling and stewing can make the difference* .... A class of toxins ..., advanced glycation end products (AGE), are absorbed into the body through the consumption of grilled, fried, or broiled animal products, such as meats and cheeses. AGEs, which are also produced when food products are sterilized and pasteurized, have been linked to inflammation, insulin resistance, diabetes, vascular and kidney disease and Alzheimer's disease."[7]

Walking After a Meal

In 2005, the *Journal of American College of Cardiology* published research that found an inverse relationship between the amount of physical activity performed and the level of ischemic stroke and coronary heart disease. Particularly, people who walked more or practiced sports more often were found to have lower rates of ischemic stroke and coronary heart disease.[8]

In 2005, the Oregon Research Institute published a research paper in the *Journal of the American Geriatrics Society* that showed blood pressure could be reduced by walking on a cobblestone mat surface. Walking on such surfaces was also found to be beneficial to adults sixty years of age and older by bettering the group's balance and physical performance.[9]

Afternoon Naps

In 2007, the *Archives of Internal Medicine* published findings from research conducted at Harvard University and Athens University that napping may reduce the risk of heart disease. From a collection of 23,681 health records of individuals ranging from the age of twenty to eighty-six with no previous history of heart disease, scientists found that people who consistently rested for a minimum of three times a week, thirty minutes or more each time, were subject to a 37 percent lower risk of dying from heart disease.[10]

The MW Institute for Chronobiology's "Sleep Cycle Distortion through Industrial Work Hours and Its Effect on Productivity and Just General Crabbiness," details a twenty-five-year study that found that "for 92.5% of workers, an afternoon nap increases their productivity, their creativity and problem solving skill."[11]

Drinking Fruit Juices

"The Power of Fruit Juice," a 2007 study by the University of Michigan, "found no association between childhood obesity and one hundred percent fruit juice." Pomegranate juice is effective in lowering low-density lipoprotein (LDL) cholesterol, the type of cholesterol responsible for causing heart disease. It "may slow the growth of prostate cancer," as well as "increase blood flow to the heart in people with ischemic coronary heart disease." Orange juice "may help prevent recurrences of painful kidney stones." Cranberry juice has long been used as a home remedy for urinary tract infections. Blueberry juice contains the same properties as cranberry juice.[12]

In 2005, the University of Wisconsin Hospital published an article indicating that citric acid reduces the formation of kidney stones.[13]

Exercising at 4 PM: Lifting Weights and Vocalization
In 1998, the Gunma University School of Medicine in Japan published a finding that "afternoon exercise improves the quality of night sleep." This research compares the effects of exercise performed during the morning and afternoon and concludes that "afternoon exercise has a better effect on sleep than morning exercise."[14]

In a 2004 interview with CNN, Dr. Phyllis Zee of Northwestern University stated, "The best time to work out is in the late afternoon. The reason for that is your muscle strength is at its peak, its highest. You're going to be less likely to injure yourself. It's also a time when people are most awake and alert."[15]

1. Weight lifting:

    In 2007, the Canadian Broadcasting Corporation (CBC) reported on joint research performed by McMaster University and the Buck Institute for Age Research, related to the effects of weight training and muscle damage. A comparative study of twenty-five healthy people in their seventies and twenty-six healthy adults in their twenties found that weight training can be used to rejuvenate the muscles of healthy, older patients in order to improve their quality of life.[16]

In 2007, CBS News reported that "exercise has type 2 diabetes benefits." A study by Canadian researchers, including researchers from the University of Calgary, found that type 2 diabetes patients must do weight lifting and aerobic exercises to improve blood sugar control.[17]

2. Vocalization during exercise (Kiai):

Kiai and Aiki are common vocalization techniques, especially in Eastern martial arts. Vocalization "relates to the coordination of one's energy with the energy emitted from an external source." In addition to advising weight lifting and vigorous exercises, Lord Liu instructed people to yell to release their frustrations. This was particularly important in the treatment of patients with addictions and mental illness.

In 2006, the *British Journal of Sports Medicine* reported on research coordinated by the University of Nevada that examined how brief yoga exercises and "motivational preparatory interventions" affected distance runners. Researchers concluded, "Motivational and yoga interventions designed to improve long distance running performance were equally acceptable to the participants, but the former [motivational shouting] had greater effect." Study subjects included ninety high school age, long-distance runners. Researchers instructed the subjects to (a) perform yoga exercises, (b) do motivational shouting exercises, or (c) do nothing, as part of the control group following a one-mile baseline run.[18]

Warm Feet Means Good Sleep

In 1999 the *Nature Journal* published a report by the Sleep Laboratory in Basal, Switzerland, that found that "you are more likely to fall asleep swiftly if your hands and feet are warmer than the temperature of the bedroom." Warming the feet can initiate the body's sleep mechanism by dilating blood vessels. Researchers performed this study on a group of healthy young men who were monitored moments before they fell asleep.[21]

In 2001, the Sleep Laboratory further reported on a direct relation between "cold feet and prolonged sleep-onset latency in vasospastic syndrome."[19] Vasospastic syndrome occurs when the blood vessels in the body either dilate or constrict in irregular ways to respond to stimuli, like having cold feet. This study indicates a correlation between having cold feet and a lengthening in the amount of time necessary for someone to fall asleep. In *Warm Feet Mean Swift Sleep*, a BBC News article explained that the dilation of blood vessels causes sleep. (Dr Kurt Krauchi and his team at the Sleep Laboratory at Basel monitored the body temperature and functions of a group of young, healthy men as they nodded off. The team found that while a hot water bottle at the feet may not directly act on the central nervous system to cause sleep, it can trigger widening of the blood vessels, which in turn switches the body's sleep mechanism on. In every case, subjects fell asleep immediately after a shift in blood flow to the hands and feet.[20]) Conversely, cold feet cause a constriction in the vessels. Vasospastic syndrome is an inherited human trait.

Spiritual Enrichment

In 2000, the *Journals of Gerontology* published a finding by the Center for the Study of Aging and Human Development at Duke University entitled "Does Private Religious Activity Prolong Survival?" The study, carried out over six years on 3,851 older adults, concludes, "Older adults who participate in private religious activity before the onset of ADL [activities of daily living] impairment appear to have a survival advantage over those who do not."[21]

In 2000, the American Psychological Association presented a study conducted by researchers, including several from the University of Alabama and the University of Santa Clara entitled, "Religious Faith and Spirituality May Help People Recover from Abuse." This study focused on 236 recovering alcoholics and drug addicts.[22]

In 2006, scientists from the University of Mississippi Medical Center presented a study concluding that "faith was linked to lower blood pressure." The study of about 5,000 African Americans monitored the effect of religious activity on diastolic and systolic blood pressure. While the study confirmed earlier research regarding the positive physiological effect of religious activity, no correlation between being prayed for and physiological effects was found. In a study of coronary bypass surgery patients, neither people for whom strangers prayed nor people for whom friends and acquaintances prayed benefited. In fact, those who knew they were being prayed for often experienced an increase in postoperative complications.[23]

Sex

Western medical studies and Lord Liu differ on the relationship of sex to health. Western studies believe that frequent sex will rejuvenate the body.

A 2002 BBC News report stated, "Frequent sex [is] not linked to strokes." BBC News based this conclusion on a University of Bristol report detailing a study of middle-aged men that found that the amount of sex a man engages in does not affect his chance of stroke. In addition, the scientists found, "Frequent sexual intercourse can actually reduce the risk of suffering a fatal heart attack."[24]

In 2007, the *New England Journal of Medicine* published research from the University of Chicago that suggested, "Frequent sex [is] linked with good health for seventy and eighty year olds." The research found that most American adults ranging from fifty-seven to eight-five years of age thought that sexuality was vital in life. Furthermore, for people who were active, the level of sexual activity only decreased by a little from the age of fifty to seventy.[25]

While modern research shows that sexual activity several times a week can contribute to leading a healthier lifestyle, there is no evidence of the benefits of refraining from this activity.

Lord Liu had a very different opinion on sexual activity. He believed that sexual intercourse was a celebration of life and creation, the most important purpose of which was the conception of a child. He recommended that men ejaculate only once a month, during their reproductive peak. By retaining their sperm, they would maximize their fertility and their offspring would be strong and healthy.

Lord Liu Chun understood that sex was a very important aspect of a human being's mental health. To maintain good mental and physical health, he encouraged couples to caress each other. This interaction was so pure and beautiful that it was compared to the textural appreciation of an exquisite jade sculpture. Lord Liu Chun thought that the human touch was vital to the emotional and physical well-being of an individual and his partner. If a woman was too ill for sexual intercourse, her partner should caress her and express his love, without engaging in intercourse. This expression of the balance between yin and yang would hasten the healing process.

In the case of eunuchs or individuals with dysfunctional sexual organs, these individuals could still satisfy natural sexual urges by caressing their wives or mistresses.

Colon Irrigation

According to ARCH, the Association and Register of Colon Hydrotherapists, in the United Kingdom, "Colon irrigation, a forty-five minute process where fifteen gallons of water gently enter the colon, is used to eliminate wastes including feces, dead cellular tissue, mucous, parasites and worms. Colon irrigation performs four main tasks: first, to clean the colon; second, to exercise the colon; third, to reshape the colon, and fourth to stimulate reflex points."[26] Groups such as ARCH and some naturopaths have advocated the effectiveness of colon irrigation, but modern Western medical doctors do not suggest colon irrigation as a useful cleansing practice.

Modern research has corroborated a majority of Lord Liu Chun's ten principles for enhancing life. Alternative or naturopathic practitioners have studied other aspects of Lord Liu's findings, including the benefits of colon irrigation. As for the remaining tenants, such as drinking one liter of fresh fruit juice daily and exercising in the afternoon, although there is little formal research on these principles, no studies have dispelled their effectiveness. The primary disparity between modern science and Lord Liu Chun's ten points is their respective beliefs as to the frequency with which men should ejaculate.

While each side of this particular debate must have its proponents, both modern science and Lord Liu Chun certainly agree that choosing a healthier lifestyle means making certain personal decisions and commitments. From one viewpoint, Lord Liu Chun's way of living is simply a collection of time-tested methods to prevent illness and enhance life.

Chapter 5
Cancer Research: Modern versus Lord Liu Chun

Historical Cancer Research in China

In 1409, the Chinese Imperial government began groundbreaking cancer research that would continue for more than thirty years. This enabled Lord Liu Chun, the head of the imperial medical staff, to develop a new and extensive method of treating cancer. The first step in the research was to stimulate the growth of cancer in death row inmates.

Researches gave two hundred female prisoners a diet of four items designed to cause deterioration of the body.

Stimulating/Creating Cancer

The inmates consumed the following substances:

- Limewater (known to cause indigestion and inflammation of the digestive tract)
- A meatless diet of rice and vegetables (to reduce protein intake and cause malnutrition)
- Toxins (three types, to create chronic inflammation, including, *Venenum Bufonius* (蟾酥, chan su); *Calomelas* (轻粉, qing fen); and *Relgar* (雄黄, xiong huang).

- Chili peppers, ginger, and leeks (According to Chinese food or nutrition therapy, food and the various methods of its preparation stimulate the yin and yang properties in the body, creating balance and imbalance. One imbalance is the production of too much heat or fire. This excess heat in the body promotes angiogenesis, the growth of new blood vessels from preexisting ones (血热妄行). If a dormant tumor is present, consuming highly stimulating foods may trigger its transformation from a dormant to a malignant state.)

After two years of these prescribed diets, these patients suffered deteriorated health. Their ailments could be categorized into four groups:

1. Breast cancer
2. Thyroid cancer, stomach cancer, and lymphatic cancer
3. Malnutrition and hemorrhoids
4. Vomiting of blood and severe difficulty in breathing

Lord Liu Chun concluded that cancer resulted from the presence of five primary symptoms in the body:

1. Bad energy in the stomach (胃气不足)
2. Malnutrition from lack of protein (吃素)
3. Genetic predisposition (胎病)
4. Toxins in the body (蓄毒内伤)
5. Excessive heat in the blood causing deviation from normal circulation (angiogenesis)

Treating Cancer

Lord Liu Chun continued his studies and repeated his methods of inducing cancer. When he had amassed a group of two hundred fifty cancer patients, he began treatment and research. He divided each group into five subgroups of fifty people. The five subgroups allowed him to focus on five separate aspects of care: overall treatment, boosting energy, correcting the blood circulation, detoxification, and pain relief.

Lord Liu and his researchers further divided each subgroup into smaller units of ten individuals. They had each unit consume a different item from a similar group of elements, in order to identify the best ingredient.

Before differentiation, all patients consumed the appetite-inducing soup, which was designed to increase their metabolism and appetite in order to maximize the absorption rate of the ingested treatment.

Herbs in Appetite-inducing Soup Given to Cancer Treatment Research Subjects

Herb Name	Latin Name	Chinese Name
guang mu xiang	*Costus* root	广木香
bei shan zha	*Fructus Gataegi*	北山楂
zhu ling	*Polyporus Umbellatus*	猪苓
hang jiu	*Chrysanthemum*	杭白菊

Note that TCM doctors use *Polyporus Umbellatus*, an herb, to reduce swelling, as it rids the body of excess water and *Chrysanthemum* to bring down the internal body heat. This concept is a traditional Chinese concept that assigns temperature to sickness or feelings such as fevers, heat stroke, inflammation or other maladies where the body will feel hot. Eating chili peppers can also increase internal heat.

In addition to ensuring that patients had an appetite, researchers gave them soup that was rich in protein. Alternating daily, patients drank freshwater fish soup and beef soup. Researchers began cancer treatment after taking these preliminary steps.

Overall Treatment:

Gallbladder has been used for centuries in ancient Chinese medicine. It is recognized as a significant element in the cure of many serious diseases.

Lord Liu used the ten-person groups to test the effectiveness of gallbladders from the following sources:

- Shark (鲨鱼胆)
- Fish (青鱼胆)
- Bear (*Fel Ursi*, 熊胆)
- Pig (猪胆)
- Chicken (鸡胆)

They found shark gallbladder to be most effective.

Correcting Blood Circulation:

In addition to the shark gallbladder, researchers administrated five types of herbs to a set of fifty new patients:

- *Radix Sanguisorbae* (地榆) (to stop internal bleeding)
- *Stigma Goci* (西红花) (to cool down the internal heat of the blood)
- *Rhizoma Chuanxiong* (川芎) (to regulate the blood)
- *Radix Angelicae Sinensis* (当归) (to nourish blood)
- Pig's liver (猪肝) (to nourish blood)

The patients who took the *stigma goci* (西红花) to cool down the blood experienced the greatest pain relief.

Boosting Energy:

Researchers gave the successful ingredients identified from two previous tests, shark gallbladder and *stigma goci* (西红花), to a new set of fifty patients in conjunction with one of the following items:

- *Radix Codonopsis Pilosulae* (党参) (to boost energy)
- *Ligum Aquilariae Resinatum* (沉香) (to cool down the internal heat and energy)
- *Fructus Awantii Immaturus* (枳实) (to correct the damaged energy flow)
- *Radix Bupleuri* (柴胡) (to divert the energy)
- *Herba Ephedrae* (麻黄) (to boost energy)

The patients in the group taking the *ligum aquilariae resinatum* (沉香) felt the most re-energized, and researchers used this ingredient in the subsequent stages of treatment.

Detoxification:

To rid the body of toxins, researchers gave a new set of fifty patients shark gallbladder, *stigma goci* (西红花), *fructus awantii immaturus* (沉香), and one of the following ingredients:

- *Rhizoma Coptidis* (黄连) (to rid dampness and the breeding of bacteria)

- *Cornu Saigae Tataricae* (羚羊角, horn of an antelope) (to get rid of wind[iii])
- *Herba Oldenlandiae* (白蛇草) (to remove blood clots)
- *Rhizoma Belam Candie* (射干) (to get rid of phlegm)
- *Flos Loncerae* (金银花) (to reduce the internal heat and fever)

The patients who consumed ground *cornu saigae tartaricae* (羚羊角) experienced the most significant recovery. The substance is derived from deer antler.

Relieving Pain:

Researchers administered a combination of shark gallbladder, *stigma goci* (西红花), *lignum aguilariae resinatum* (沉香), and *cornu saigae tartaricae* (羚羊角) to a new set of fifty patients, in conjunction with one of the following pain-relieving ingredients:

- *Radix Notoginseng* (参三七) (to stop bleeding)
- *Radix Stephaniae Tetnandrae* (防己) (causes urination to rid the body of excess water and reduce swelling and inflammation)
- *Radix Angelicae Dahwricae* (白芷) (to reduce wind)
- *Bornpolam Syntheticum* (冰片) (to rid the body of internal heat)
- *Lindera Aggregate* (乌头) (to cause drowsiness; the Chinese administered this herb during surgical procedures)

---

iii   In TCM, wind has a few characteristics: (1) Wind tends to float. Thus, wind causes disease that involves the surface of the body, the head, and the face and manifests as headache or runny nose. (2) Wind tends to move. It causes tremor of limbs, dizziness, spasm, or convulsion. (3) Wind tends to change. Wind causes disease characterized by a sudden onset and immediate transmission.

The patients who took the first ingredient, *radix notoginseng* (参三七), experienced the greatest pain relief.

After many years of exhaustive experimentation, Lord Liu Chun concluded from his studies that the most effective treatment for cancer was a medicine consisting of:

- Shark gallbladder (鲨鱼胆)
- *Stigma Goci* (西红花)
- *Ligum Aguilariae Resinatum* (沉香)
- *Cornu Satigae Tartaricae* (羚羊角)
- *Radix Notoginseng* (参三七)
- A group of ingredients that has been kept as a Liu family secret

This combination of ingredients seemed to cure cancer in the patients, but it caused undesirable side effects. Lord Liu and his researchers recognized that the dried powder form of the shark gallbladder caused uncontrollable vomiting and diarrhea. After many years of investigation, the researchers found a solution to this problem. They placed the shark gallbladder in rice vinegar for five years, and the result was a detoxification of the gallbladder and elimination of the negative side effects.

Another challenge arose from the initial studies. Lord Liu Chun found that, although the breast cancer patients were cured of breast cancer, some patients suffered from cancer that had metastasized to other parts of the body. Researchers could not find a solution, until they identified a patient whose cancer had not metastasized. The researchers studied her diet and lifestyle for insight into her body's ability to prevent metastasis. As the wife of a butcher, she had enjoyed a diet rich in protein and had consumed large quantities of her favorite food: bovine tendon (牛筋).

Lord Liu Chun investigated the matter, and after twenty years of research, he substantiated that there was a correlation between bovine tendons and the prevention of cancer. In particular, the tendon contained inside the hoof (deep flexor tendon), has the greatest density, and Lord Liu Chun and his descendents proved it to be the most effective treatment for stopping cancer from metastasizing or spreading. The idea is that the collagen in the tendon wraps around and encloses the cancer cells, which prevents them from growing. For those who subscribe to the belief that cancer cells are present in everyone's body (remaining dormant in some), collagen type 1 is preventative; it envelops the dormant cells and prevents them from growing. This therapy is unique because the treatment is the same for all cancers. Lord Liu Chun also identified similar tendons in horses, camels, bears, and mules.

Bovine tendons became a staple in the cancer research study, and Lord Liu and his team finalized the formula to treat cancer as follows:

1. Soup composed of *radix aucklan dial* (guang mu xiang 广木香), *fructus gataegi* (bei shan zha 北山楂), *polyporus* (zhu ling 猪苓), and *Chrysanthemum* (杭白菊) for detoxification and stimulation of appetite
2. Protein soup (freshwater fish and beef)

3. Shark gallbladder (鲨鱼胆)
4. *Stigma goci* (西红花) to cool down the blood
5. *Ligum aguilariae resinatum* (沉香) to balance energy
6. *Cornu saigae tartaricae* (羚羊角) to get rid of excess wind
7. *Radix notoginseng* (参三七) to stop bleeding and relieve pain
8. Other catalytic ingredients that are kept secret by the Liu clan[iv]
9. *Kong yan san* (控岩散)
10. Tendon soup made from the deep flexor tendon

Lord Liu Chun's thorough research was critical to the imperial family. In 1454, Empress Zhou (周淑云皇贵妃) was diagnosed with breast cancer. Lord Liu Chun applied his cancer treatment methods and cured the empress. She was able to prolong her life by forty-two years and died of old age.

Shark Gallbladder

Historical Chinese Research

Nine hundred years ago, in the twelfth century, an ancestor of Lord Liu Chun, Dr. Liu Wansu (刘元素), found that shark gallbladders could be used in the treatment of cancer. Lord Liu Chun used shark gallbladders when he treated the Empress Yong Le. The treatment prolonged her life by seven years, and she died in 1407.

Fresh shark gallbladders, however, caused many side effects, including diarrhea, vomiting, and a loss of appetite. Lord Liu and his researchers corrected this problem by soaking the gallbladders in rice vinegar for five years.

---

iv   Items 3 through 8 are the ingredients of Lord Liu's cancer medication.

Lord Liu Chun also discovered that shark gallbladder, when used singularly as treatment, was not sufficient in inhibiting the spread of cancer. To keep the cancer from spreading, he combined the gall bladder with four other ingredients: *Stigma goci* (西红花), *Ligum aguilariae resinatum* (沉香), *Cornu saigae tartaricae* (羚羊角), and *Radix notoginseng* (参三七). In addition, Lord Liu discovered that deep flexor tendons in the Achilles tendon were crucial in the prevention of the spread of cancerous tumors.

Western Research

Squalamine is an aminosterol compound (a steroid substance) found in the bile-producing organs, such as the liver and gallbladder, of the dogfish shark.

> Dr. Michael Zasloff first identified squalamine in July 1993. Zasloff was particularly interested in the immune systems of sharks. He worked with Karen Moore, a medical student, in a search for antibiotics that are produced in nature. Initially, Zasloff and Moore conducted this research hoping to find a treatment for infection. Dr. Zasloff performed another study for the National Academy of Sciences in 1993 on the aminosterol antibiotic qualities of squalamine from sharks.[1]

In the 1990s, Dr. Henry Brem researched squalamine looking for characteristics that would help in the fight against breast cancer. Dr. Brem found that squalamine affected blood vessel proliferation (angiogenesis), the process by which tumors nourished themselves by creating circulatory paths.[2]

Another team of scientists led by Dr. Richard Pietras of the University of California, Los Angeles, was working to isolate the traits of squalamine. This team found that squalamine was antiangiogenic in ovarian cancer xenografts and that the compound had the ability to enhance the cytotoxic effects of cisplatin on ovarian cancer cells .This finding revealed that squalamine had the ability to inhibit the growth of blood vessels in an ovarian tumor and to render the cancer cells more susceptible to the chemotherapy drug cisplatin.

Researchers have performed many more studies in the effort to identify the chemical benefits of squalamine, as recognition of this animal product's potential importance has fueled heightened interest in it. In 2001, the Lombardi Cancer Center of the Georgetown University Medical Centre in Washington, DC, and Magainin Pharmaceuticals (currently Genaera Corporation, in Plymouth Meeting, Pennsylvania) performed a "phase I and pharmacokinetic study of squalamine, a novel antiangiogenic agent, in patients with advanced cancers."The study is to determine the maximum tolerated dose, dose-limiting toxicity of the squalamine.[3]

Magainin Pharmaceuticals teamed up with the Cancer Therapy and Research Center of the Institute for Drug Development in San Antonio, Texas, to conduct another study in 2001, which found that "squalamine treatment of human tumors in nu/nu mice enhances platinum-based chemotherapies."[4] The two tests described above prove that medical researchers have taken an interest in the squalamine drug as an anticancer treatment, and later studies, such as the trial listed below, show that modern medicine recognizes it in the treatment of cancer.

In 2003, the University of Texas, the Institute for Drug Development, Cancer Therapy and Research Center in San Antonio, Texas, and Vanderbilt University in Nashville, Tennessee, reported on "a phase I/IIA trial of continuous five-day infusion of squalamine lactate (MSI-1256F) plus carboplatin and paclitaxel in patients with advanced non-small cell lung cancer."[5] Researcher administered squalamine to forty-five patients for five days, in combination with the chemotherapy drugs, palitaxel and carboplatin, on the first day, to test the toxicity of the combination. They found that patients could safely ingest this combination and that squalamine should be further explored for its effectiveness as a complement to chemotherapy.

Lord Liu Chun's prescription suggests a less harmful way to use squalamine without the damaging effects of chemotherapy. In addition, Lord Liu's formula calls for paclitaxel extracted from the yew tree; traditional Chinese medicine has documented the use of paclitaxel in its natural form. The chemical drugs used in cancer treatment by Western medical professionals are potent and harsh on the body. Lord Liu Chun's methods will take more time in terms of how soon the treatment will take effect, but they harvest ingredients in their natural form, making them safer to use.

The presence of squalamine in shark gallbladder substantiates Lord Liu Chun's visionary use of this ingredient in his remedy for cancer. Nevertheless, researchers should continue to study squalamine further. So far, its effectiveness has been tested in three primary applications: (1) as an antibiotic, (2) in the field of cancer research, and (3) in the study of age-related macular degeneration (AMD).

Squalamine was also a key ingredient in the FDA-approved drug EVIZON, a treatment for AMD, but with the formulation of more effective treatments and products, EVIZON is no longer on the market.

Squalamine occurs naturally in sharks, and Western scientists have been trying to produce a synthetic replacement. In 2006, the Department of Chemistry at Lehigh University in Bethlehem, Pennsylvania, and the Infectious Disease sector of the Harvard Institute of Medicine published research results in a n article called "A Bioconjugate Approach Toward Squalamine Mimics: Insight into the Mechanism of Biological Action."[6] This study shows that scientists can effectively synthesize squalamine in small amounts while preserving its original antibacterial properties.

In 2003, the Niigata University of Pharmacy and Applied Life Sciences researched the synthesis of squalamine from desmosterol.[7]

In 2000, Dr. Michael Zasloff patented the "treatment of carcinomas using squalamine in combination with other anti-cancer agents" (US Patent 6147060).[8] Commercial interest in other aspects of cancer research thwarted Dr. Zasloff's attempts to fund further research, but in recent years, clinical trials for cancer and eye disease are providing further information about squalamine.

A medical company in New Zealand published findings in 2004 stating, "A new product, Ketsuge, developed by a Melbourne scientist, is based on Isolutrol (sodium scymnol sulphate) from shark bile, and was found to control the skin's oil production."[9]

In 2005, French scientists wrote a review titled "Squalamine: A Polyvalent Drug of the Future?" The article speaks of the benefits of squalamine and its potential drug use in the future. Among the benefits of squalamine are its abilities to aid in the treatment of cancer, age-related macular degeneration (AMD), and weight gain.[10]

Collagen Type I (骨胶原1类) in Deep Flexor Tendon of the Achilles Tendon

Historical Chinese Research

With the development of *kong yan san*（控岩散, the Liu family remedy that combines shark gallbladder, four herbs commonly prescribed in Chinese medicine—*Stigma goci* (西红花), *Ligum aguilariae resinatum* (沉香), *Cornu saigae tartaricae* (羚羊角), and *Radix notoginseng* (参三七)—and other herbs that remain a family secret, Lord Liu Chun and his researchers had finally formulated an effective treatment for cancer, and this treatment has cured many patients.

In one group of patients, although the treatment eradicated the original cancer, metastasis occurred. Lord Liu Chun conducted trials with many different herbs and medicines, but he could not stop the relocation of cancer cells. He observed that, in one particular patient, the cancer had not metastasized. As mentioned earlier, this patient was the wife of a butcher, and her favorite food was bovine Achilles tendons. Lord Liu Chun considered the possible connection between the woman's full recovery from cancer and her consumption of the bovine Achilles tendon.

For more than twenty years, Lord Liu Chun researched and experimented with the tendons in his search for a definitive cure for cancer. He found that the deep flexor tendon in the bovine Achilles tendon did indeed prevent the spread of cancer. The tendons were the necessary ingredient to complete the cancer treatment, as they provided a method for preventing metastasis. They complemented the primary ingredient, shark gallbladder, which was vital to the cure of cancer (岩者，食牛筋而安).

Western Research: What Exactly Is Bovine Achilles Tendon?
Zimmer Dental Inc. released a statement about their product BioMend, an absorbing wound dressing, which indicates that the active ingredient in the product is bovine Achilles tendons. Zimmer Dental wrote, "Bovine Achilles tendon is known to be one of the purest sources of Type I collagen that can be readily obtained and processed in commercial amounts."[11]

In 2007, Obihiro University of Agriculture and Veterinary Medicine in Japan released a research paper entitled "Some Bovine Proteins Behave as Dietary Fibres and Reduce Serum Lipids in Rats." The article commented on the effects of both bovine Achilles tendon and artery proteins and their similarities to dietary fibers. Researchers It was found that particular forms of protein could act as dietary fibers and reduce serum lipid concentration "by enhancing faecal neutral sterol excretion or suppressing lipid synthesis in the liver."[12]

In 2006, Ehime University and Marutomo Co. Ltd. published research titled "Immunostimulation Effect of Jellyfish Collagen." The paper stated that "purified collagen from bovine Achilles tendon accelerated IgM production of hybridoma cells. These facts mean that collagen has an immunostimulation effect ...."[13]

Type I collagen is found in the tendons, and it has been recognized by various authorities as an effective inhibiting material applicable in many uses due to its polymerizing characteristics and ability to self-assemble.

In another article, "Collagen Deposition on a Preformed Grid," a team of scientists from the University of Hawaii and the University of Colorado mentioned the useful characteristics of collagen. They wrote, "The fine filaments [of a matrix material] may be self ordering, extracellular macromolecules which in turn determine the polymerization of collagen fibrils."[14] The *Journal of Materials Chemistry* also published a paper about "films of self-assembled purely helical type I collagen molecules," which comments on the polymerization characteristics of collagen.[15] These two studies demonstrate the unique self-assembly capability of collagen type I.

In 2002, the American Society for Investigative Pathology submitted a paper to the *American Journal of Pathology* entitled "New Approaches to the Biology of Melanoma." This research repeatedly cited results from DeClerk Laboratory studies about of the role of the extracellular matrix in melanoma proliferation. The paper attributed the specific use of collagen type I to the "inhibitory effect (...) specific to type I collagen and was "not observed in the presence of other ECM proteins such as laminin, fibronectin or vitronectin."[16] The researchers then observed two forms of collagen type I, natural and denatured, *with regards to the impermeability of the matrix.* They concluded, "When present in an intact fibrillar form, type I collagen exerts a negative effect on cell proliferation, whereas when denatured or proteolyzed, it has a positive effect."[17]

In the 2001 *Proceedings of the National Academy of Science of the United States of America*, "Integrin Activation Controls Metastasis in Human Breast Cancer" discusses an experiment in which researchers employed collagen I from bovine tendons to create a matrix in blood vessels. Researchers measured the arrest of breast cancer cells during blood flow and the way the cells interacted with platelets. They found, "Briefly, tumor cells were suspended in human blood and perfused over a collagen I matrix at a venous wall shear rate. Adhesive events and cell interactions were visualized."[18] Venous blood returns to the heart (in veins), and wall shear rate (WSR) is the derivative of blood velocity with respect to vessel radius. What these researchers found, then, is that the collagen type 1 matrix interacted with the tumor cells. This isn't a conclusion that the collagen type 1 could stop breast cancer, but it is an indication that the collagen matrix interacted with, arrested, and suspended the tumor cell.

In 2007, a breakthrough study from the National Cancer Center Research Institute in Tokyo, Japan, reported, "Type I collagen gene [in humans] suppresses tumor growth and invasion of malignant human glioma cells."[19]

Lord Liu Chun originally documented the idea of orally ingesting collagen for therapeutic purposes more than six hundred years ago. In recent years, many researchers have explored a similar approach. In 2005, a group of universities including Johns Hopkins issued the following information about their test results: "A unique treatment approach uses collagen from cows (oral type 1 collagen) that the patient eats. It is based on the idea that the immune system is more tolerant of digested foreign proteins than those detected in circulation. Once patients consume the collagen, researchers hope that the body will produce T-cells that recognize the cow's collagen as harmless and will then suppress the attack that is occurring on the patient's own, similar, collagen."[20] Many studies found that bovine collagen did appear to help the immune system of scleroderma patients become more tolerant of their own collagen.[21]

Western research indicates that, if type I collagen can create a matrix, it can arrest the cancer cells. However, if the matrix is denatured or deformed, the cancer cells will grow upon the matrix and spread even more.

Dr. Liu Hong Zhang (Lord Liu Chun's twenty-fourth descendant) has observed that his ancestor's treatments for cancer have limited efficacy under certain conditions:

1. The patient has no appetite despite having received the appetite-inducing soup.
2. The patient has previously received radiation treatment or chemotherapy.
3. The patient suffers from acute leukemia.

Conclusion

Bovine Achilles tendon is one of the purest forms of type I collagen. This type of collagen can reduce the amount of lipids (fats) in the body and boost the immune system. Type I collagen can also prevent cancer cells from spreading by enveloping them. Type I collagen is present in the skin, bones, and tendons, but the Liu family only uses the bones and tendons of cows to enclose cancer cells. According to Chinese medical theory, consumption of animal skin increases the body's ability to retain fluid and, thus, increases swelling and pain in cancer patients.

The research cited on previous pages indicates that the denaturation of type I collagen will cause cancer cells to spread even faster. We may hypothesize that, when a cancer patient undergoes operation, radiation, or chemotherapy, the treatment is considered a success if the treatment eradicates all the cancer cells. If cancer cells remain, there is a possibility that they will spread at an accelerated rate because the type I collagen cells have been damaged and cannot inhibit cancer cell growth.

Modern research and theory explains many of Lord Liu Chun's practices. One vital aspect still remains to be examined: the medical efficacy of type I collagen ingested orally as soup. In Dr. Liu Hong Zhang's experience, the X-rays of many patients who consumed soup prepared from the deep flexor tendon of the bovine Achilles tendon for at least three months showed a characteristic change in cancerous tumor shape. Their cancer tumors were transformed from irregular shapes to more rounded ones. In some cases, simply drinking the soup caused the tumors to shrink in size by preventing sporadic growth. This is an area of research and a scientific breakthrough that modern medicine needs to explore.

In the fifteenth century, Lord Liu Chun had never heard of type I collagen. Through observation of a patient who did not develop cancer after a variety of cancer-inducing trials, he discovered the effectiveness of the deep flexor tendon in the bovine Achilles tendon. Lord Liu developed a soup that facilitated the digestion and absorption of the collagen through the simmering of the tendon for twelve hours. He was not aware of the self-polymerizing traits of the tendon. Despite this lack of modern technology and scientific proof, he was able to identify the remarkable characteristics of the tendon.

In the last ten years, Western research has proven the effectiveness of bovine Achilles tendon but has not developed a universal technique to deliver type I collagen as medication in order to inhibit the spread of cancer cells.

Albert Einstein once opined, "The development of Western science is based on two great achievements: the invention of the formal logical system (in Euclidean geometry) by Greek philosophers, and the discovery of the possibility to find out causal relationships by systematic experiment (during the Renaissance)." According to Einstein, "One has not to be astonished that the Chinese sages have not made those steps. The astonishing thing is that those discoveries were made at all."[22]

When a patient requires immediate emergency relief, surgical procedures, immunization, or analysis of disease (急救，防疫，手术，病理诊断), Western methods are more effective. It is commonplace today for a Chinese practitioner to request medical attention from a Western doctor if surgical procedures, X-rays, blood analyses, or infant delivery are required. It is equally common for a Western doctor in China to seek the medical attention of a Chinese practitioner for chronic diseases.

The National Cancer Institute has stated, "Bovine cartilage and shark cartilage have been studied as treatments for cancer and other medical conditions for more than thirty years."[23] The research of Lord Liu Chun and his descendants has finally been translated, in order to draw parallels between Eastern and Western schools of thought in the quest to cure cancer. The Chinese methods date back six hundred years and have been kept secret as treatment exclusive to the Imperial court, but now it is time to reveal the secret and share with the world many years of study and knowledge.

Physicians in China have used Lord Liu Chun's prescribed shark gallbladder and deep flexor tendon of the bovine Achilles tendon to treat cancer for over six hundred years. Lord Liu Chun and his descendants have successfully treated many patients historically, and they continue to do so today. As admirers who have personally witnessed the effectiveness of Lord Liu Chun's methods, we welcome the scientific study of Lord Liu Chun's ideas and treatments. We encourage more detailed research of the methodology to find the correlation between modern science and historical proof. Although the concept of food therapy has existed for many centuries, it is still not widely accepted. The Nobel Prize awarded in 1934 to researchers of liver therapy was a turning point in the history of modern medicine.

In time and with additional research, food therapy will become a more accepted practice that can be used in every household.

Current Application of Lord Liu Chun's Methods

Today, Dr. Liu Hong Zhang, Lord Liu Chun's twenty-fourth descendant, is applying Lord Liu's traditional methods of treating chronic diseases. Before treatment, Dr. Zhang advises patients to undergo Western medical examinations such as blood tests, urine tests, and magnetic resonance imaging (MRI) or X-ray. He currently instructs cancer patients to follow the steps listed below:

1. Consume Appetite-inducing soup, which consists of:
   - 100 grams bei shan zha (北山楂, Hawthorn fruit)
   - 50 grams guang mu xiang (广木香, *Costus* root)
   - 50 grams *Chrysanthemum* (杭菊)
   - 50 grams zhu ling (猪苓, *Polyporus umbellates*)

   To relieve pain, patients or caregivers can add the following ingredients:

   - 100 grams jin yin hua (金银花, Lonicera japonica Thunb)
   - 20 grams cao jue ming (草决明, Catsia tora Linn)

   To relieve coughing, patients or caregivers can add another set of ingredients:

   - 10 grams ma huang (麻黄, Herbal Ephedrae)
   - 10 grams gan cao (甘草, Radix Glycyrrhiza)

2. Consume deep flexor tendon soup.

Deep Flexor Tendon Soup

1 pound deep flexor tendon[v]

2 liters cold water

0-50 grams bei shan zha (optional)

0-10 dried red dates (optional)

> (1) Add tendon to a pot of cold water and bring to a boil.
>
> (2) Reduce heat and simmer for twelve hours, making sure to repeatedly skim the. fat.
>
> (3) Add bei shan zha and dried red dates for additional flavor.

This soup is very rich and can cause nausea and diarrhea in patients who have insufficient hunger. (See the section in Chapter 3, entitled "Preparing Appetite-Inducing Soup.") If refrigerated, the soup will congeal into a gelatinous substance. For cancer patients who suffer from large tumors, the preparer may use a larger portion of tendon. The patient should decide how much tendon to use, based on his or her ability to digest. The amount can vary from a half pound to two pounds of tendon, prepared in one to two liters of water. You can also combine the soup with one or both of the other two soups and use it as stock for cooking noodles or vegetables.

3. Avoid eating seafood. Seafood is rich in iodine, which is believed to cause the dispersal of tumors in the body.

---

v   Lord Liu Chun's original prescription is based on the use of the deep flexor tendon of the bovine Achilles tendon (in the hoof of the animal). This provides the best source of collagen type 1. If the deep flexor tendon is not available, you may substitute with the superficial flexor tendon of the Achilles tendon (commonly available in supermarkets), but results are superior with the deep flexor tendon.

4. Avoid eating chili peppers or any spicy food.
5. Abstain from drinking any alcoholic beverages.
6. Refrain from smoking tobacco.
7. Maintain a calm disposition.
8. Avoid constipation. To make a natural laxative, grind fifty grams of raw sesame and combine it with water to form an edible paste.
9. Abstain from strenuous exercise or sexual intercourse.
10. Follow Lord Liu's philosophy of the enhancement of life. Colon cancer patients should omit the steps regarding colonic irrigation.
11. After the patient has consumed soup made from the deep flexor tendon of the bovine Achilles tendon for three months, the cancer should be enclosed and might not enlarge further. This is the time to begin a course of kong yan san, the Liu family remedy for cancer prevention. The dosage varies, depending on the patient. Patients under the age of fourteen, over the age of seventy, or weighing less than fifty kilograms should not exceed three capsules, four times a day. Patients outside these parameters can use up to five capsules, four times a day. As treatment progresses and cancer tumors become smaller and denser, patients may experience prolonged, uncomfortable pain. The kong yan sang dosage can be reduced slightly, but the patient must eat more appetite-inducing soup to boost metabolism. When fully recovered, the patient must continue to take a minimum dose over his lifetime to prevent reoccurrence of the illness, since Lord Liu has classified genetic predisposition as one of the five causes of cancer.

Unlike other cancer treatment plans whose first step is *taking medicine*, the Liu family's treatment plan calls for first *rekindling the appetite* with appetite-inducing soup and *encapsulating the cancerous cells* with tendon soup.

Western researchers studying the benefits of squalamine need to be mindful of this tendency for patients to feel increased discomfort as the tumor tissues become smaller but denser. The dosage of medication might also need to be adjusted.

Over the past six hundred years, the Liu family has upheld a strong religious devotion to Buddhism and maintained good relationships with Buddhist monks. The family, which has practiced medicine for the past nine hundred years, has observed that Buddhist monks rarely succumb to cancer; however, if a monk does develop cancer, his return to health is a very difficult process. Due to their vegetarian diet, monks are deficient in animal protein. They respond very slowly to appetite-inducing soup and are reluctant to drink the bovine Achilles tendon soup. Often, their digestive systems have been so conditioned to years of meat-free diet that their bodies reject the soup. Through years of involvement in the Buddhist community and the observations described above, the Liu family discourages a vegetarian lifestyle.

During any healing process, patients should seriously consider Lord Liu's ten points to the enhancement of life. No amount of treatment can be effective if the patient indulges in a lifestyle that is contraindicative.

Chapter 6
Diabetes: Lord Liu's Historical Research Versus Modern Research

Historical Diabetes Research in China

In 1409, the Chinese Imperial government approved a thirteen-year research project on diabetes. This enabled Lord Liu Chun, the head of the imperial medical staff, to develop a new and extensive method of treating diabetes.

His first step was to induce the symptoms of diabetes. Again, he used inmates on death row. He gave two hundred inmates a diet of limewater, vegetarian food, and sugar water, a diet designed to cause rapid deterioration of the body. Then, after administering appetite-inducing soup, Lord Liu systematically sought out the best decoction for treating the diabetes.

Induction of Diabetes
Lord Liu knew that limewater caused indigestion and inflammation of the digestive tract. In addition, he gave the inmates a meatless diet of rice and vegetables to reduce the amount of protein they consumed, causing malnutrition. He also prescribed sugar water.

After six months, some inmates showed diabetic symptoms such as thirst, hunger, and persistent urination (their urine attracted ants, which indicated that it had a high sugar content). Lord Liu Chun concluded that diabetes resulted from the presence of four main symptoms in the body:

1. Bad energy in the stomach
2. Malnutrition from lack of protein
3. Genetic predisposition
4. Deficiency of yin energy causing internal heat （阴虚内热）

Lord Liu Chun continued his studies and repeated his process of inducing diabetes. When he had amassed a group of two hundred diabetic patients, he began another cycle of treatment and research.

Treatment of Diabetes

Lord Liu gave all patients the appetite-inducing soup, which was designed to increase their metabolism and appetite in order to maximize the rate of absorption of the substances he was analyzing.

In addition, he gave the patients soup rich in protein. Alternating daily, patients drank freshwater fish soup and beef soup.

After these preliminary steps, Lord Liu began the diabetes treatment. He divided the two hundred inmates into twenty groups of ten people. He gave each group a different decoction of the substances listed below:

Decoctions Tested in Order to Find Treatment for Diabetes

Group	Decoction	Latin Name	Chinese Name
1	gou qi	*Fructus Lycii*	枸杞汤
2	ma huang	*Herba Ephedrae*	麻黄汤
3	xiao hui xiang	*Fructus Foeniculi*	小茴香汤
4	ren shen	*Radix Ginseng*	人参汤
5	jin yin hua	*Flos Lonicerae*	金银花汤
6	zhi shi	*Fructus Auranti Immaturus*	枳实汤
7	ci shi	*Magnetitum*	磁石汤
8	sha shen	*Radix Glehniae*	沙参汤
9	wu mei	*Fructus Mume*	乌梅汤

10	di yu	*Radix Sanguisorbae*	地榆汤
11	dang gui	*Radix Angelicae Sinensis*	当归汤
12	zhu ling	*Polyporus Umbellatus*	猪苓汤
13	Jing Jie	*Herba Schizonepetae*	荆芥汤
14	qing huo	*Rhizoma Seu Radix Notoptery-gii*	羌活汤
15	chuan bei mu	*Bulbus Fritillariae Cirrhosae*	川贝母汤
16	mu li	*Concha Ostreae*	牡蛎汤
17	cao jue ming	*Cassla Tora L*	草决明汤
18	chuan xiong	*Rhizoma Ligustici*	川芎汤
19	bei shan zha	*Fructus Crataegi*	山楂汤
20	shi jun zi	*Fructus Quisqualis*	使君子汤

After one month, the researchers noted that three groups exhibited reduced diabetic symptoms. They were groups 5 (*Flos Lonicerae,* 金银花), 8 (*Radix Glehniae,* 沙参), and 18 (*Rhizoma Ligustii,* 川芎).

Lord Liu Chun combined the medicines from these three groups and made a special decoction with them. Most patients improved, although a few showed no change in their conditions.

Lord Liu Chun studied the patients who had not improved and discovered that they had bribed their prison guards with money for extra rice and alcohol. After eliminating the banned food and continuing to drink the medicinal decoction, the patients recovered.

Improving Circulation

Lord Liu removed the inmates who no longer suffered from diabetes from the research project, and prison administrators released them on the northern border of China. Later, some of them suffered from blood clots. Lord Liu Chun sought a remedy to improve circulation. This led to another series of tests on two hundred patients.

Lord Liu's objective was to develop a formula to nourish the body and help the body retain fluid. Chinese medicine had already identified certain foods for their effective properties. The following table lists the foods Lord Liu served to each group in this experiment.

Foods and Herbs Tested in Order to Find
Formula for Improving Blood Circulation

Group	Food/ Herb	English/Latin Name	Chinese Name
	wu mei	*Fructus Mume*	乌梅
	sheng di	*Rehmannia Glutinosa Libosch*	生地
	e jiao	*Colla Corii A sini*	阿胶
	huang ming jiao	N/A	黄明胶
	hai shen	*Holothuria* (sea cucumber)	海参
	hai zao	*Sargassum*	海藻
	shan yu rou	Common *Macrocarpium* fruit	山萸肉
	yang cai	Watercress	洋菜
	fu pen zi	*Fructus Rubi*	覆盆子
	shan yao	*Dioscorea Opposite*	山药
	huang lian	*Rhizoma Coptidis*	黄连
	xuan shen	*Radix Scrophulariae* (fig-wort root)	玄参
	xi jiao	(Rhinoceros horn)	犀角
	shi gao fen	(Gypsums powder)	石膏粉
	bai he	*Bulbus Lilii*	百合
	tian hua fen	*Radix Trichosanthis*	天花粉
	he li le	Medicine *Terminalia* fruit	诃黎勒
	zhu pi	(Pork skin)	猪皮
	niu pi	(Beef skin)	牛皮
	yang pi	(Sheep skin)	羊皮

In Groups 18 and 19, after several days of consuming pig and beef skin, patients no longer felt the constant thirst symptomatic of diabetes.

Zheng He (郑和), China's Greatest Sea Explorer (1371–1435)
When Zheng He was twelve years old, he was castrated and entered the imperial palace to begin a lifelong service as a eunuch. Emperor Yong Le favored him for his intelligence, eventually promoting him to

the rank of admiral and giving him command of 317 ships and 27,800 soldiers. Zheng He traveled as far as East Africa and the Arabian Peninsula. On Zheng He's sixth trip, he realized that he constantly felt thirsty and needed to urinate, both indicators of diabetes. Due to the water rations onboard ship and his self-imposed limit of two liters of water a day, Zong He was very thirsty and uncomfortable.

In 1422, upon his return to China, he went to Nanjing to seek help from Lord Liu Chun. Since Lord Liu and Zheng He were good friends, Lord Liu was aware of Zheng He's habit of drinking copious amounts of sweetened tea to maintain vigilance.

After thirteen years of researching the cure for diabetes, Lord Liu had developed a new medicine called *Han Xiao Shan*. He gave this medicine to Zheng He and instructed him to follow a three-pronged treatment:

1. Eliminate sweetener from his tea
2. Drink appetite-inducing soup and beef skin soup (instead of pork skin because Zheng He was Muslim)
3. Follow a course of treatment with the new medicine, *Han Xiao Shan*

After a month, Zheng He arrived unexpected at Lord Liu's home and immediately ordered him to kneel. Lord Liu thought that somehow he had incensed the emperor and was about to be punished. Then, Zheng He jokingly chastised him for withholding such a useful cure and allowing so many people to suffer from diabetes. Zheng He encouraged Lord Liu to manufacture for sale to the public a jelly made from porcine or bovine skin soup. Lord Liu, however, felt that the ingredients were easily accessible and that the recipe should not be proprietary.

The table below lists the main ingredients in *Han Xiao Shan*. Lord Liu used this prescription to cure diabetes six hundred years ago, and it has been a well-known and often-used treatment since then.

The Ingredients in Han Xiao-Shan

Chinese Name		Latin Name
龟板	gui ban (turtle shell)	*Plastrum Testudinis*
鳖甲	ao jia	*Carapax Trionycis*
鱼鳔	yu biao	*Isinglass*
紫稍花	zi shao hua	Freshwater Sponge *Spongilla*
西红花	xi hong hua	*Stigma Croci*

Lord Liu Chun's medicine, *Han Xiao Shan*, contains five principal ingredients, two of which are derived from turtle shell, *Plastrum Testudinis* (龟板) and *Carapax Trionycis* (鳖甲). Lord Liu discovered that the carbonate and alkaline properties of the shell could balance the acidity associated with diabetes.

Three severe complications known to result from diabetes are diabetic ketoacidosis, hyperglycemic hyperosmolar state, and lactic acidosis.[1] Twenty years ago, sodium bicarbonate was used as treatment for diabetes. Currently, the medical community is debating this chemical's efficacy. Nevertheless, both Lord Liu Chun and more recent pharmaceutical manufacturers have relied on formulae with an alkaline base in their treatment of diabetes.

While the turtle shell is not a proven source of sodium bicarbonate, Professor Donald Jackson of Brown University documented a similar neutralizing effect in 2000. Dr. Jackson's report provides information that corroborates Lord Liu's decision to treat the acidity of diabetes with turtle shell. "Anoxic turtles accumulate high levels of lactate in blood. To avoid fatal acidosis, turtles exploit buffer reserves in their large mineralized shell. The shell acts by releasing calcium and magnesium carbonates and by storing and buffering lactic acid."[2]

Conclusion

Through exhaustive examination and thorough testing of food combinations, Lord Liu Chun concluded that the formula for curing diabetes consisted of avoiding starch and alcohol, drinking the appetite-inducing soup, drinking the soup made from pig or beef skin, and taking the medicine, *Han Xiao San* (函消散). In the twentieth century, Lord Liu Chun's twenty-second descendant, Dr. Liu Feng Chi (刘凤池), successfully used this technique to cure Taiwanese president Jiang Jie Shi (蒋介石).

Elastin and Collagen Treatment from Pork and Beef Skin Soup

Western Research

According to Western medicine, the skin is composed of three layers: the epidermis; the dermis; and the subcutaneous tissue. The thickest layer is the dermis, composed mainly of collagen and elastin. The body's production of these substances declines with age. This explains how a child with youthful, elastic skin gradually becomes an adult with wrinkles and sagging skin.[3] The modern world's obsession with the preservation of a youthful appearance has fueled many a laboratory's race to discover the most effective formula to replenish lost elastin and collagen through topical creams and lotions.

Although we may ridicule beauty cream manufacturers and dismiss their claims that elastin and collagen revitalize our skin, we might be surprised to learn that beauty—and the effects of elastin and collagen—is truly more than skin deep. Research completed over the last twenty years consistently emphasizes that elastin and collagen play important roles in diabetes, respiratory disease, and heart disease.

In 1997, the Department of Biology and Immunology of the University School of Medicine in Bulgaria published research entitled "Elastin Peptides as a Marker of the Severity of Vascular Complications in Diabetes Mellitus." Researchers reported, "Elastin is one of the main proteins in the vascular wall and elastin degradation is accelerated in diabetic patients."[4] The American Diabetes Association is idea was also explored this idea in a 2003 report on how elastic and muscular arteries age. This report concluded, "There are significant differences in the rate of age-related decline in vascular stiffness in elastic arteries of nondiabetic compared with diabetic arteries." We can infer that the arteries of diabetics have lost more elastin and are less elastic than those of their nondiabetic peers.[5]

The importance of elastin in the understanding of respiratory diseases can be found in the following research: In 2000, the *American Journal of Respiratory Cell and Molecular Biology* published "Impaired Distal Airway Development in Mice Lacking Elastic." This report indicated, "Elastin is a major component of the mammalian lung, predominantly found in the alveoli. Destruction of alveolar elastic fibers is implicated in the pathogenic mechanism of emphysema in adults. This data defines the role of elastin in the structure and function of the mature lung and suggests that elastin is important for alveogenesis."[6]

A 2006 publication by the American Physiological Society again highlights the significance of elastin in the body. This report, "Lungs Try to Repair Damaged Elastic Fibers," articulates the importance of elastin in the respiratory system and indicates that the lungs of juvenile emphysema patients try to repair themselves after damage. Finding a method to facilitate this could enable the regeneration of new alveoli and result in a decrease in the mortality rate associated with emphysema.[7]

In 2008, Apria Healthcare published the following information about chronic obstructive pulmonary disease: "In emphysema, there is permanent destruction of the alveoli, the tiny elastic air sacs of the lung, because of irreversible destruction of a protein in the lung called elastin that is important for maintaining the strength of the alveolar walls. The loss of elastin also causes collapse or narrowing of the smallest air passages, called bronchioles, which in turn limits airflow out of the lung. The number of individuals with emphysema in the United States is estimated to be 2 million."[8]

Researchers have also named elastin as an important factor in the study of heart disease. A 1998 Howard Hughes Medical Institute article suggests that loss of elasticity in arteries may accelerate heart disease. The report states, "In the arterial system, where the protein is most abundant, elastin forms an elastic mortar between the arrays of cells that line the arteries."[9]

We can infer that elastin is vitally important in the composition of the human body, particularly with regards to the maintenance of healthy lungs and arteries. Deterioration of lungs and arteries can lead to respiratory and heart disease, as well as diabetes.

The excerpts from modern medical research are a small sample of the studies that are currently ongoing with respect to collagen and elastin. What is equally fascinating is the scientific examination of collagen, elastin, and the presence of these substances in the skin of humans and animals.

In 2005, the *Journal of Histochemistry and Cytochemistry* published "Multiple Roles for Elastic Fibers in the Skin." This article states, "Dermal elastic fibers are believed to have a primary role in providing elastic stretch and recoil in the skin." It also comments on the elastin content (specifically desmosine, a special amino acid that comes from four lysine residues and is found only in elastin) of skin in different animals (note that a picomole [pmol] is one-trillionth of a mole, a standard unit of measurement that designates the number of things [usually atoms or molecules] in an experiment or study):

> Most animal skin contained from one hundred to three hundred pmol desmosine/mg protein. The human skin used in this study was from an 8-month-old child and was significantly higher in elastin content than the other animals, which had a value of six hundred pmol desmosine/mg protein. ... The elastic fibers did not present as long fibers or align in organized sheets as was observed with human skin. Unlike other animals investigated, with the exception

of human, the majority of the elastic fibers in pig skin did not appear to originate from cells lining hair follicles and did not show the normal network of elastic fibers surrounding the follicle in the upper dermis. ... In human skin, and to a lesser degree, pig skin, the elastic fibers lie as parallel fibers in the entire depth of the dermis.[10]

Western scientists are currently culturing pig skin as an effective treatment of open burn wounds.[11]

Elastin is found abundantly in the skin, blood vessels, and lungs, but it is only produced in humans under the age of thirteen or fourteen. Patients suffering from diabetes, cardiovascular disease, respiratory disease, and mental illness exhibit reduced elastin levels. While treating diabetics, Dr. Liu Hong Zhang found that drinking pig skin soup produced two results: a decrease in blood sugar levels and a decrease in nighttime urination. Patients with heart disease and high blood pressure experienced a decrease in blood pressure. In theory, he recognized the health benefits of elastin, but the actual amount of elastin transferred into the body by edible forms is subject to debate. More research is needed in this area.

Lord Liu's Research

Six hundred years ago, Lord Liu Chun was already aware of the significance of pork and beef skin. Although he preferred pork skin, he examined the use of beef skin as an alternative treatment for China's large Muslim population.

Lord Liu Chun's methods offer the natural replenishment of the body's store of elastin through the consumption of animal-based ingredients. Lord Liu Chun found that patients who had consumed porcine or bovine skin exhibited lower blood pressure and reduced diabetes-related symptoms. (As with Lord Liu Chun's treatment for cancer, we hope that researchers will investigate further and document the connection between the results and their underlying scientific explanations.)

When Lord Liu was developing a treatment for diabetes, he noted that patients who drank the soup containing liquefied pork or beef skin experienced reduced likelihood of stroke and frequent urination. He found that pork or beef skin soup benefited patients who suffered from any of four major illnesses:

- Diabetes
- Cardiovascular disease
- Respiratory conditions
- Mental illness

Patients who suffered from these conditions would follow three steps of treatment:

1. Appetite-inducing soup to invigorate metabolism
2. Pork or beef skin soup
3. Herbal medicine:

   - For diabetes: *han xiao san* (函消散)
   - For cardiovascular disease: *tong xuan san* (通玄散)
   - For respiratory problems: *na qi san* (纳气散)
   - For mental illness: *zhi mi san* (指迷散)

The first two steps—appetite-inducing soup and pork/beef skin soup—are crucial to the treatment of any patient. They are the hallmark of Lord Liu's approach to the prevention of illness and represent the idea of "seven parts nurturing." Ingesting medicine or consuming nutritious food is not effective when the body is so weak that it cannot absorb medicine or nutrients and is vulnerable to foreign bacteria.

Perhaps Lord Liu Chun's method of simmering pork or beef skin for twelve hours to extract the elastin, collagen, and other properties is a more natural and efficient way of replacing these lost substances than attempting to reintroduce them medicinally. It is possible that this liquefied elastin and collagen is easier to absorb and distribute throughout the body than topical applications.

Current Treatment

Today, Lord Liu Chun's twenty-fourth generation descendant, Dr. Liu Hong Zhang, applies Lord Liu's traditional methods of treating chronic diseases. Before any treatment, Zhang advises his patients to undergo Western medical examinations, such as blood tests, urine tests, MRIs or X-rays, as these methods are diagnostically superior to traditional Chinese testing methods.

Zhang currently uses the following technique to treat diabetes patients:

1. Stimulate appetite with appetite-inducing soup:
   100 grams bei shan zha (北山楂, Hawthorn)
   50 grams guang mu xiang (广木香, *Costus* root)
   50 grams *Chrysanthemum* (杭菊)
   50 grams sha shen (沙参)

2. Drink pork or beef skin soup for nutrition
   Pork or Beef Skin Soup
   1 pound skin, fat removed[vi]
   2 liters cold water
   0-50 grams bei shan zha (optional)

---

vi   Use pork or beef skin that has had the underlying layer of fat removed or, if skin is not available, substitute with two pounds of pig trotters. Pig trotters contain a great amount of fat, and the resulting soup must be repeatedly skimmed or chilled to remove the fat.

0-10 dried red dates (optional)

(1) Add skin or trotters to a pot of cold water, bring to a boil, and simmer for twelve hours.
(2) Add bei shan zha and dried red dates for additional flavor.

This soup is rich in soluble, easily digested elastin. If refrigerated, it will congeal into a gelatinous substance. You can combine the soup with fish or beef soup. If you're using pig trotters, be sure to discard the meat.

3. Avoid consumption of chili pepper or stimulating herbs.
4. Adopt Lord Liu Chun's ten steps to the enhancement of life.
5. Complete prescribed treatment of *han xiao san*.

Note: Diabetes patients tend to feel hungry. While testing the effectiveness of various herbs, Lord Liu Chun noticed that, when diabetes patients drank only two liters of water a day, they did not feel hungry. The patients only experienced hunger, a false hunger, after drinking water to compensate for their frequent urination. Six hundred years ago, Lord Liu Chun advised diabetes patients that they must rekindle their appetites in order to regain their health.

Chapter 7
Food Is Medicine

Lord Liu Chun recommended consuming one liter of soluble protein soup (pork skin, bovine tendon, beef, or freshwater fish soup). He also recommended drinking one liter of fresh fruit juice and consuming a diet rich in fiber and fresh vegetables.

He tested his theories on patients and determined that food contains therapeutic properties that need to complement a patient's health profile. One man's medicine could be another man's poison. Below are some of the examples he noted:

- People suffering from constipation should avoid spinach.
- Those with high blood pressure should avoid pumpkin, as it increases blood pressure.
- Mango promotes coagulation of blood. Menstruating women should avoid consumption in order to avoid the formation of ovarian cysts (子宮肌瘤).
- Certain foods are diuretic, and people with diabetes and/or high blood pressure should avoid them. Diuretic foods cause the blood to thicken and increase the production of urine. These include coffee, tea, celery, lettuce, winter melon, watermelon, kiwi, pineapple, strawberries, and grapes.

- Cancer patients should avoid bamboo shoots, onions, peaches, and chestnuts because they stimulate blood circulation and cause metastasis of cancer cells.
- Cancer patients should also avoid lemons, as they cause water retention and swelling.
- Cancer patients and patients suffering from high fever should avoid pig skin soup because it causes water retention and swelling.
- Cancer patients should further avoid lychee, walnut, lamb, goose, and squab because they are very nourishing and will promote rapid growth of any existing tumors.
- Cancer patients should avoid seafood and seaweed, which are high in iodine. Iodine dissolves phlegm and causes existing tumors to divide and spread.
- Finally, cancer patients should avoid peanut, water chestnut, pomello, and kumquat also dissolve phlegm. These foods will cause existing tumors to divide and spread.

Western research initiated over the last two decades has also focused on the therapeutic effects of vegetables, fruit, and their juices. A 2003 study by the University of California Irvine Medical Center in Southern California evaluated the antibacterial properties of various fruit and vegetable extracts on common potential pathogens including antibiotic-resistant strains. Green vegetables showed no antibacterial activity on *Staphylococcus epidermidis* and *Klebsiella pnemoniae.* Purple and red vegetables and fruit juices had antibacterial activities in dilutions ranging from 1:2 to 1:16.[1]

In 2004, Japanese researchers at the Department of Pharmacy of the Miyazaki Medical College Hospital examined how star fruit potently inhibited human cytochrome P450 3A (CYP3A) activity. CYP3A are enzymes that metabolize a wide variety of xenobiotics (any substances that are foreign to living systems), including drugs.

Because CYP3A are localized in both the liver and the intestine, they can contribute to presystemic elimination of substrate drugs after oral administration (first-pass metabolism). Relying on the results, researchers hypothesized that, like grapefruit, the filtered extracts of star fruit could alter pharmacokinetics of therapeutic drugs co-administered via CYP3A inhibition. In other words, star fruit or its juice may hinder the metabolism process. Thus, the possibility of the adverse food-drug interaction by the star fruit or star fruit juice with medicine through CYP3A metabolism should be examined in vivo.[2]

Yet another study was conducted in August 2006 on the effects of fruit. Researchers from the University of Alabama School of Medicine and the DCH Regional Medical Center in Alabama studied the management of grapefruit-drug interactions. Prominent medications known to interact with grapefruit include statins, antiarrhythmic agents, immunosuppressive agents, and calcium channel blockers.[3]

The US Cancer Institute recommends that patients eat peanut butter[4], but traditional Chinese medicine presents an opposing view. According to Chinese medicine, peanuts have the ability to disperse phlegm. In a similar manner, the consumption of peanuts may have the ability to cause cancer to metastasize.

In 1433, the Minister of Defense, Xu Kuo (许廓), died at the age of sixty-six. The minister was from Sichuan province and enjoyed eating spicy foods, in particular, water-boiled fish (水煮鱼). This dish contains hot chili, many spices, and a large quantity of oil. The minister consumed it almost every day and, coincidentally, suffered chronic migraines. Xu Kuo served as minister for only a year and a half until his death.

Lord Liu Chun wondered about this incident and how the minister's eating habits might have contributed to his early demise. He sent an undercover soldier to serve as a chef in a restaurant. After a few weeks, the soldier was able to report on how chefs prepared this dish. They used freshwater fish, but the soup contained more than seventy ingredients.

Lord Liu Chun made some speculations on the minister's death based upon his eating habits. The minister had unknowingly filled his body with substances that were medically contraindicative and harmful. Lord Liu Chun's analysis of the ingredients found them to include the following properties:

- Aphrodisiac (壮阳类中药)
- Stimulating (热性类中药)
- Energy-enriching (保气类中药)
- Heat-lowering (清热类中药)
- Enriching of the yin energy (滋阴类中药)
- Preventing diarrhea/constipating (止泄类中药)
- Blood-coagulating (止血类中药)
- Phlegm-dissolving (化痰类中药)
- Antibacterial (杀虫类中药)
- Containing a large amount of sugar (高糖高热量 类中药)

The minister's favorite dish contained an overwhelming amount of strong ingredients, as well as copious amounts of salt and sugar that further upset the delicate balance of his body. It caused indigestion and internal bleeding in the stomach.

Lord Liu Chun believed in consuming simple, unprocessed, and unrefined foods such as fruits and fruit juice, vegetables, food with high fiber, and protein soup. He preferred taking large quantities of protein soup over a diet heavy in solid meat.

Based upon his ancestor's practice and his own experience, Dr. Liu Hong Zhang has listed some common health problems and their food-related origins:

A child appears tired or unable to concentrate after eating

The child's food contains monosodium glutamate and meat-based artificial flavoring additives. These chemicals negatively affect a child's delicate nervous system.

A child is feverish. The fever subsides with fever-reducing medicine, but it returns when the medicine wears off.

The child may be consuming food and beverages high in processed sugar. The sugar in ice cream, chocolate, candy, and baked snacks over-energizes the body and causes increased body temperature.

A pneumonia patient completes his treatment of medication but continues to suffer from a persistent cough.

He is eating spicy, oily food that irritates the esophagus and trachea.

A patient suffers from persistent diarrhea.

She continues to consume fatty meat.

A cancer patient drinks the bovine tendon soup to retard further cancer cell growth yet still experiences metastasis of cancer cells.

The soup is being prepared with stimulating seasonings such as ginger, pepper, garlic, and green onions.

A bronchitis patient follows his course of medical treatment but appears to still suffer from his illness.

He eats foods that contain excessive amounts of vinegar and sugar.

A patient with a sore throat finishes her course of treatment but still has a sore throat.

She likes to eat food with chili, pepper, and ginger.

A diabetic adheres to his prescribed medical treatment but still suffers from a high blood sugar level.

He drinks large amounts of tea, coffee, and carbonated beverages containing large amounts of sugar.

When we eat, our purpose should be to provide nutrients for our body. We should eat to live, not live to eat. If we are driven by taste only, we will very easily succumb to illness.

Many of the Qing dynasty emperors practiced healthy eating habits and enjoyed good health. In the royal palace, the imperial chefs relied only on a limited palate of ingredients including sesame sauce, sweet paste, dates, Hawthorn berries, radish, brown sugar, salt, and tomato paste. Their vegetables were grown organically on a royal farm where they were irrigated by spring water from Jade Fountain Hill near Beijing. All live fish, before consumed, were put in clean water for a few days.

The emperors took breakfast around 7:00 AM, a heavier mid-day meal at 12:00 PM, and a very light snack at 6:00 PM.

There were three imperial kitchens: the tea kitchen, the bakery kitchen, and the main kitchen. Except for special occasions, the emperor had his meal alone.

The imperial family did not live as lavishly as one would have expected. Despite the exquisite meals and exotic foods available to them, they did not indulge in such extravagances on a daily basis and, instead, limited their consumption to try to maintain long and healthy lives.

Chapter 8
Lord Liu Chun's Food Therapy

The Origin of Meat and Fish Soup

Lord Liu Chun embarked on a quest to identify the most nutritious and most easily absorbed food suitable for all age groups. This food would strengthen the body, support the immune system, and prevent illness. On his quest for this superfood, he conducted hundreds of experiments on multiple groups of two hundred inmates.

Initially, he gave two hundred inmates only appetite-inducing soup for seven days. The subjects were greatly weakened by their hunger and lack of nourishment. The first food that the inmates consumed after a week of appetite-inducing soup was either a liquid nutrient or a nutrient in pureed form. Lord Liu then divided the inmates into twenty groups of ten people; each group consumed one of the following individual foods:

Nutrition from vegetables

Corn	Rice	Wheat noodles
Glutinous rice	Soy beans	
Millet	Soy bean milk	

Nutrition from annimals (puree or liquid)

Beef	Boiled eggs (10)	Duck
Chicken	Dog	Mutton
Cow's milk	Donkey	Pork

Nutrition from the ocean and lakes (puree)

Freshwater fish	Squid and octopus
Sea cucumber	Turtle

Lord Liu repeated this "first food" experiment multiple times using hundreds of food types. He observed that subjects who had consumed ground beef and freshwater fish experienced the most improved health and strength.

Lord Liu carried out another series of experiments to find the best cooking method for the identified ingredients and the optimum quantity of each ingredient. He divided a new group of two hundred inmates into twenty subgroups of ten.

Researchers simmered one pound of ground beef in one liter of water for two hours. They duplicated the same cooking method in ten test cases. In each case, they extended the cooking time by two hours. Thus, Group 1 consumed soup from one pound of beef simmered in one liter of water for two hours, and Group 10 consumed the same quantity simmered for twenty hours.

Alternately, researchers simmered the same quantity of beef in two liters of water and, again, extended the cooking time by two-hour increments. Thus, Group 11 consumed soup from one pound of beef simmered in two liters of water for two hours, and Group 20 consumed the same quantity simmered for twenty hours.

Documentation showed that the inmates in Group 16 were the first to regain their strength and health. From these results, Lord Liu concluded that beef soup simmered for twelve hours in two liters of water achieved the best patient recovery.

Interestingly, the results were identical when researchers used freshwater fish as the primary ingredient in the soup. The difference was the freshwater fish soup benefited people with acute diseases, while the beef soup was more beneficial for patients suffering from chronic diseases.

Soup and Memory

Lord Liu Chun continued his experiments on the beneficial properties of soup and the affects of nutrition on health. He called for one hundred and eighty middle-aged inmates, who were divided into six groups of thirty. He gave each group a set diet and instructed them to memorize and recite a different article daily.

1. Group 1 ate lean beef. Within twelve months, all the inmates had developed delayed responses.
2. Group 2 ate lean beef, rice, and potatoes every day. After only six months, the group had developed delayed responses.
3. Group 3 ate lean beef, millet, and potatoes every day. After eighteen months, this group began experiencing delayed responses.
4. Group 4 ate beef soup. Researchers never observed signs of delayed, even after twenty-four months.
5. Group 5 ate beef soup, rice, and vegetables. After twenty-four months, this group began to experience delayed responses.
6. Group 6 ate beef soup, foods high in fiber, and potatoes. Researchers observed no signs of delayed response, even after twenty-four months.

After repeating this experiment in several trials, Lord Liu concluded that a diet of solid meat and little fiber was harmful to the body and the mind. People needed to consume protein soup and foods high in fiber to maintain good health.

Different Protein Soups

Freshwater fish soup is crucial to patients suffering from acute illnesses. This soup is rich in nutrients and easy to absorb.

Ground beef soup is good for treating chronic illnesses. Alternating between these two soups is another option for patients who are chronically ill.

Cancer patients should drink soup made from the deep flexor tendon of the bovine Achilles tendon, as well as freshwater fish and ground beef soups. Cut up the tendon during the cooking process to facilitate liquefaction.

Patients with diabetes or cardiopulmonary problems should drink soup made from pork or beef skin with the underlying layer of fat removed. Cut up the skin during the cooking process to facilitate liquefaction. To minimize fats and oil, skim while simmering or remove fat after refrigeration.

Patients suffering from anemia should eat pork or beef liver, as well as blood tofu (血豆腐) made from the blood of pigs, cows, ducks, or chickens.

People who are healthy and do not suffer from any major illness can drink *Boyuan* soup (保元汤) to maintain good health. The recipe is provided in this chapter.

All the soups can be used as bases for congee, wonton, or noodles. You may add vegetables such as tomatoes, turnips, carrots, and potatoes at the end of the cooking time.

The method for preparing soup is described below.

1. Simmer for twelve hours.
2. Avoid all spices except salt or soy sauce. Never add stimulating spices such as ginger, garlic, onions, or pepper.
3. Skim animal fat and oils from the soup.

4. If using an electric slow cooker, maintain the temperature on a low setting.
5. For flavoring, add an optional 50 grams of bei shan zha and ten small red dates. *Do not add any other herbs.*

Recipes for Meat and Fish Soups

Freshwater Fish Soup

2 pounds whole fish, cleaned, descaled, and gutted

2 liters cold water

0-50 grams bei shan zha (optional)

0-10 dried red dates (optional)

Fish soup is made from freshwater fish. Do not use saltwater fish, as it contains iodine.

Remove innards and scales. Add the entire raw fish, including head and tail, to two liters of cold water and simmer for twelve hours. For flavor, you may add bei shan zha or dried red dates. After twelve hours, one liter of soup should remain. Remove and discard the fish carcass. You may add vegetables at the end of the cooking period. This soup can be used as stock for dumplings, pasta, or vegetable soup.

Ground Beef Soup

1 pound lean ground beef

2 liters cold water

0-50 grams bei shan zha (optional)

0-10 dried red dates (optional)

Add beef to a pot of water and simmer for twelve hours. For additional flavor, add bei shan zha and dried red dates. The resulting soup is a soluble protein that is easily absorbed. You may removed and discard the meat before serving. If adding vegetables, add them at the end of the cooking period. This soup can be used as stock for dumplings, pasta, or vegetable soup.

Deep Flexor Tendon Soup

1 pound deep flexor tendon	Lord Liu Chun originally prescribed using the deep flexor tendon of the bovine Achilles tendon (in the hoof of the animal). This provides the best source of collagen Type I. If the deep flexor tendon is not available, substitute the superficial flexor tendon of the Achilles tendon (commonly available in supermarkets). However, results are superior when the deep flexor tendon is used.
2 liters cold water	
0-50 grams bei shan zha (optional)	
0-10 dried red dates (optional)	

Add tendon to a pot of cold water, bring to a boil, reduce heat, and simmer for twelve hours. Repeatedly skim the fat. Add bei shan zha and dried red dates for additional flavor. The amount can vary from a half pound to two pounds of tendon, prepared in one to four liters of water. You may combine the soup with one or both of the other two soups and use it as stock for cooking noodles or vegetables.

If cancer patients suffer from large tumors, use more tendon to prepare the soup. The patient should decide how much tendon to use based on his or her ability to digest.

Pork/Beef Skin Soup

1 pound skin, fat removed[vii]

2 liters cold water

0-50 grams bei shan zha (optional)

0-10 dried red dates (optional)

(1) Add skin or trotters to a pot of cold water, bring to a boil, and simmer for twelve hours.

(1) Add bei shan zha and dried red dates for additional flavor.

This soup is rich in soluble, easily digested elastin. If refrigerated, it will congeal into a gelatinous

---

vii   Use pork or beef skin that has had the underlying layer of fat removed or, if skin is not available, substitute with two pounds of pig trotters. Pig trotters contain a great amount of fat, and the resulting soup must be repeatedly skimmed or chilled to remove the fat.

substance. You may combine it with fish or beef soup.

If using pig trotters, be sure to discard the meat.

Beef tendon soup is also useful for the following medical conditions: influenza, cold sores, thin nasal membrane, hepatitis, urinary tract infection, post-surgery healing, wounds, burns, sports-related muscle injuries, hernia, and hemorrhoids.

Pork skin soup is useful as a blood thinner, to prevent heat stroke, and to nourish the vocal chords. It is offered to reduce perspiration during sleep and to treat bed-wetting, erectile dysfunction, asthma, and prematurely aging skin. Do not administer it under conditions of influenza, fever, or water retention.

Liver for Anemia

Pig's liver or cow's liver can be sautéed in a small amount of cooking oil. Patients on a soft-food diet can eat pureed liver or blood tofu made from the blood of pigs, cows, chickens, or ducks. This may cause some indigestion, and the patient's stool will be darkened.

Patients suffering from anemia should eat a minimum of a half pound of either liver or blood tofu daily until hemoglobin levels increase. Generally, one month of treatment is required to raise hemoglobin levels effectively.

Boyuan Soup （保元汤）

Zhang Xiang Zhai (张祥斋) was the last to serve as head eunuch during the Qing dynasty. He was born in 1876 and died in 1957 at the age of eighty-one. He was a longtime friend of the Liu family.

In 1956, Liu Shi Kai (刘世奎), Dr. Liu Hong Zhang's father, took his ten-year-old son, Hong Zhang, to Tianjin to pay his New Year respects to the old eunuch.

Liu Hong Zhang was always curious about the functions of a eunuch's genitals (since castration was a mandatory prerequisite of the profession), but he was forbidden from asking any impolite questions. When Liu Hong Zhang finally met the eunuch, he was shocked to see such a handsome man. The young boy stared in awe at the eunuch's smooth skin, youthful appearance (Zhang Xiang Zhai had no age spots), and healthy features. He was awestruck by the seemingly eternal youth of the eunuch, who was approaching the venerable age of eighty years. Overcome by his curiosity, young Hong Zhang wondered if the eunuch had used many skin creams. Zhang Xiang Zhai laughed and asked the boy if he had ever drank the very soup developed by the Liu family centuries ago. Liu Hong Zhang's father had to explain that, under political persecution by the communist movement of Mao Ze Dong (毛泽东), the Liu family had been ridiculed as examples of outdated nepotistic tyranny and traditional Chinese medicine (医霸). The family had been forced to set aside their practices, including that of preparing Boyuan soup.

During the Qian Long （乾隆） era of the eighteenth century, Liu Liang Yu （刘良玉）, the fourteenth-generation descendant of Lord Liu Chun, became the imperial physician. He offered Boyuan soup to the emperor.

> Boyuan soup contained only five ingredients:
> 1 pound freshwater fish
> ½ pound minced beef
> 1 pig's trotter
> 0-50 grams bei shan zha (Hawthorn) (optional)
> 0-10 dried red dates (optional)

Imperial physicians simmered the soup for twelve hours then skimmed the animal fat and oils. They served it during the morning, afternoon, and evening meals to immediate members of the imperial family (emperors, empresses, imperial concubines, princes, and princesses). From that point on, the soup was a staple in the imperial palace for two centuries.

Eunuch Zhang Xiang Zhai, however, nearly lost his life over the soup. One summer, Empress Dowager Cixi (慈禧太后) drank the soup and developed diarrhea and nausea. Convinced that there was a plot to poison her, she ordered the arrest and execution of Eunuch Zhang. The empress called upon the imperial physician, the twentieth-generation descendant of Lord Liu Chun, Liu Xuan Ji (刘璇玑), to cure her illness. Dr. Liu did not think that the soup had caused the problem, since he had sampled it himself. Dr. Liu found that the Empress Dowager had drunk a pear soup the previous night and diagnosed that soup as the true cause of her illness.

Eunuch Zhang was exonerated, and he remained forever indebted to the Liu family for saving him from an early execution.

In 1909, as head eunuch, Eunuch Zhang recommended the twenty-first-generation descendant of Lord Liu Chun, Liu Lian Zhong (刘连 仲), to President Yuan Shi Kai (袁世凯) as personal physician.

In 1913, at the end of the Qing dynasty, Eunuch Zhang retired from palace life and bought a house surrounded by many parcels of land in Tianjin, where he lived with his four wives. At the time of his death in 1957, he was eighty-one years old and still in excellent health. Eunuch Zhang chose to end his own life in protest of the confiscation of his possessions.

Cooking Methods Can Make a Difference

In April 2007, researchers at the Mount Sinai School of Medicine published a study on how cooking methods can impact disease. A press release announced, "Study Shows Food Preparation May Play a Bigger Role in Chronic Disease than was Previously Thought." The researchers noted, "Steaming, boiling or making stews can make a difference. Keeping the heat down and maintaining the water content in food reduces AGE level."[1] Scientists believe that AGEs (advanced glycation end products) cause many chronic and age related diseases such as diabetes.

The finding that cooking stews slowly is beneficial corroborates Lord Liu Chun's recommendation to simmer the soups for twelve hours. Slow cooking is a healthy cooking style that most effectively renders nutrients into an easily absorbable state.

Liver Therapy

At the beginning of the twentieth century, researchers made two groundbreaking discoveries in the medical field. The first was insulin; the second was liver therapy.

In 1934, George R. Minot and William P. Murphy of the Harvard Medical School and George H. Whipple of the University of Rochester School of Medicine and Dentistry received the Nobel Prize for their work with liver therapy treating anemia.

The trio gave patients with anemia 120 to 240 grams of cooked beef liver; 120 grams of mutton "muscle meat"; and various amounts of vegetables, fruits, eggs, and milk. The scientists studied the resulting red blood cell count and noticed an increase.

Whipple initiated this study in 1920 in an attempt to investigate the influence of food on blood regeneration; the rebuilding up of the blood; and, with anemia, the loss of blood.

In his experiments, Whipple caused dogs to bleed so that they had insufficient amounts of blood. Whipple tried different types of foods and found the most efficient source that would regenerate the blood cells to be liver, followed by kidney, then meat, and finally some vegetables and fruits like apricots.

Prior to these results, the medical community generally believed that large doses of arsenic would stimulate red blood cell manufacturing; blood transfusion or removal of the spleen were also standard practices. It seemed highly unlikely that food could have such astounding effects as medicine. Even now, in the age of pharmaceuticals, it is amazing to recognize the healing power of food. An excerpt of Professor I. Holmgren's1934 Nobel Prize presentation speech commending the efforts of Whipple, Minot, and Murphy reads, "It is quite a strange conception, and one lying remote from the customary beat, that came into the minds of Minot and Murphy, when they bethought themselves, that it might possibly be feasible to treat a patient suffering from this disease by administering food to him."[2]

In another passage of the speech, Holmgren states:

As consequently there was nothing that could with any degree of certainty be expected to result from the application of the diet in question, and as the method of treatment demanded such unreasonably large quantities, it is clear that the experimenters must of necessity have been possessed of an extraordinary measure of far-sightedness, an extraordinary degree of energy and an extraordinarily clear grasp of all the circumstances of the case, as they were enabled to succeed in inducing the patients to submit to such a regiment notwithstanding its disagreeableness.

If Minot and Murphy had not been imbued with such an irresistible urge to bring matters to a head, so to say, their discovery would never have been achieved.[3]

Holmgren comments on the interest with which he observed medical science's reaction to this altered aspect of the matter, referring to those who adhere to "*quasi-medical*" or "*medico-religious bodies*" and who suggest that medical science is a type of religion or philosophical system, based upon irrefrangible tenets that do not allow of alteration or modification.

The presenter goes on to say, "It is in fact a quite common disease (pernicious anaemia), for instance, it is estimated that, previous to 1926, the year in which Minot's and Murphy's methods of treatment were first applied, about six thousand persons died of pernicious anaemia every year. I have calculated—very approximately—that, since the date when their methods began to be generally applied, some fifteen or twenty thousand persons must have been saved from death in the United States alone."[4]

With the aid of modern technology and global initiatives, we can extract and preserve food's healing attributes to create compact cures for easy digestion and absorption. During the 1934 Nobel Prize Awards ceremony, Professor I. Holmgren, a member of the Royal Caroline Institute, commented, "Even after the composition of the blood had been restored by the liver treatment to a normal state, it was obligatory to make the patients continue to eat large quantities of liver, in order to keep up their recovered health. During the years that have elapsed since then, the technique of the treatment has undergone development: the active agent or stimulating substance in the liver has been successfully extracted, an extract being thereby obtained that contains the active substance in a more concentrated form."[5]

Hippocrates, the father of Western medicine, said in the times of ancient Greece, *"Thy food is thy medicine, thy medicine is thy food."* Six hundred years ago, Lord Liu Chun realized that anemia could be cured using beef liver, pig liver, and blood jelly. Additionally, Lord Liu Chun discovered the benefits of fish soup for acute diseases, beef soup for chronic diseases, bovine flexor tendon soup to inhibit the spread of cancer tumors, and pork or beef skin soup as a supplement toward curing diabetes, cardiovascular problems, and mental illness.

Lord Liu Chun performed sixty-six years of intensive experiments on death row inmates, and for the past six hundred years, Lord Liu Chun's descendants have cured millions of sick patients.

We are keen to share this information with the international medical community in the hope of perpetuating Lord Liu Chun's mission to make his remedies available for everyone.

Chapter 9
Chinese Herbal Medicine

The Use of Chinese Herbal Medicine

Chinese herbal medicine has existed for millennia, and its efficacy has been debated for an equally long time. Today, some form of herbal medicine is being used in more than one hundred and thirty countries. One hundred and twenty of those countries have established research facilities to study the remedies by analyzing their ingredients and their effects. Western research methods are being applied to certify Chinese herbal medicine. In "Patent Protection for Chinese Herbal Medicine Product Invention in Taiwan," researcher Jerry I. H. Hsiao refers to a survey revealing that 60 percent of anticancer drugs and 75 percent of the anti-infectious drugs approved from 1981 to 2002 were of natural origin. In addition, Hsiao reports that sixty-one of all new chemical entities discovered in that period were inspired by natural products.[1] What is interesting about the nature of such drugs is that the plants and natural entities cannot be patented for use. Pharmaceutical companies either synthesize or modify the structure of the natural product. By adding some form of mechanical improvement, such as purification, companies are able to patent the drugs for commercial and economic use. They preserve the positive attributes of the natural product, while altering the structure of the product to make it patentable.

According to a World Health Organization (WHO) estimation, 80 percent of the world's population uses herbal medicines as the principal form of health care. The approximately five thousand plants used in Chinese herbal medicine are the primary source of medical treatment for 90 percent of the rural population and 40 percent of the urban population in China. The WHO further states that a quarter of all prescription drugs used in Western medicine can be said to have components that originate from plant life. Aspirin is one such drug; it contains compounds that were first found and extracted from *Salix alba*, a willow tree, and *Filipendula ulmaria*, the herb meadowsweet. Quinine (金鸡纳碱/奎宁), an antimalarial drug, was first used by Jesuit priests who used the bark of *Cinchona ledgeriana*, a tree with origins in South America.[2]

The use of herbal medicine has been documented throughout history, but its efficacy comes under severe scrutiny due to a lack of communication and comprehension. Many researchers may perform clinical tests on these herbs, but few have publicized their findings. This low rate of publication is especially apparent when contrasted with the publication frequency of researchers who pharmaceutical companies fund to develop new prescription drugs. The popularization of alternative medicine in Western culture has resulted in gradual steps toward a greater reliance on herbal medicine. In 1988, Norman Farnsworth of the University of Illinois published an article entitled "Screening Plants for New Medicines." Farnsworth commented on the lack of interest in new programs for discovering drugs from plants. "What really seems to be the problem is that most pharmaceutical firms, as well as decision-making offices in government agencies, lack personnel who have a full understanding and appreciation of the potential payoff in this area of research."[3]

Farnsworth also mentions the medical community's ongoing discussion of the value of herbs as a cure for cancer: "The National Cancer Institute in the United States has tested 35,000 species of higher plants for anticancer activity. Many of these have shown reproducible anticancer effects, and the active principles have been extracted from most of these and their structures determined. However, none of these new drugs have yet been found to be safe and effective enough to be used routinely in humans."[4]

In 2007, researchers at King's College of London, England, explored the vast field of herbs used in Chinese medicine hoping to discover chemical compounds that could form the basis of pharmaceutical drugs. An astounding 8,000 chemicals were taken from the most popular 240 Chinese herbs to be tested in this extensive, revolutionary research. A database has been created for all the uses of these plants, which include ginseng, gingko, cloves, and mint. Of the 240 herbs tested, more than 62 percent are thought to be capable of curing a single disease, while more than 50 percent could potentially be applicable in the cure for two or more diseases. The very possibility of a cure could be in nature, the root of existence.[5]

Extraction of Herbs

Lord Liu Chun was very surprised at the results of his experimentation with herbs on death row inmates. He discovered that ingesting arsenic rock powder (砒石) was less toxic than ingesting an extract of the same substance (砒霜). He also found that the Chinese liquor Er Guo Tou (乌头酒) is more toxic than guo tou itself and that chan su (蟾酥) is more poisonous than toad skin (蟾皮). He concluded that nonnatural substances derived from chemical extraction became more potent than the naturally occurring forms (提炼之物，并非天合，在故其毒甚也).

We now live in the age of pharmaceuticals. Researchers are analyzing the chemical properties of herbs to develop herbal extractions that can be mass produced.

A perfect extract is very difficult to obtain. The herb itself may contain vitamins, fiber, protein, carbohydrates, sugars, oils, and many other elements that are destroyed during the chemical process. Let's consider our fruits and vegetables. Have we succeeded in producing safe extracts of fruits or vegetables with the same nutritional value as the unprocessed ingredient? So far, scientists have not been able to produce futuristic food capsules using natural food and its properties. In health food stores, one can buy various extracts of natural food such as gingko and Echinacea. However, only a portion of the natural ingredients' properties are present in the extracts.

Chinese herb formulae are most often composed of an array of different herbs that are simmered in liquid. During the simmering, many chemical reactions take place that modern technology has not successfully identified. Although Chinese doctors may use a basic formula in treating an illness, the quantity of each herb prescribed is customized to suit the patient. Currently, the American Food and Drug Administration (FDA) has not issued any approvals of Chinese medicines.

Despite the aid of modern technology, the process of herbal extraction will continue to be of limited success. The only feasible method would be to condense Chinese medicine into capsules after the herbs have been simmered in liquid. This process is similar to that used in the preparation of food for the astronauts. Instead of taking pills in lieu of fruits and vegetables, the astronauts eat dehydrated food.

Toxicology and the Validity of Herbs

In 1407, Empress Yong Le died of breast cancer. As Emperor Zhu Di mourned the loss of his beloved spouse, he transferred her responsibilities to Imperial Concubine Wang, who managed the royal palace and gradually gained the admiration of the emperor and his court. In 1421, she suddenly fell ill and would not eat. The imperial physician was summoned, and he prescribed ma huang xi xin fi zi decoction (麻黄细辛附子汤), containing *Radix Aconiti Praeparate* (附子), *Herba Ephedrae* (麻黄), and *Herba Asari* (细辛).

There was no improvement in Concubine Wang's condition. Her body was very cold, and her muscles became spasmodic. The imperial physician then prescribed si ni decoction (四逆汤), containing *Radix Aconiti Praeparate* (附子), ginger, and *Radix Glycyrrhizae* (甘草). Imperial Concubine Wang passed away that evening. She was forty-one years old.

Emperor Zhu Di was extremely angered by the deaths of these two beloved women. The imperial physician and his family were executed.

Over time, a rumor that other palatial concubines had poisoned Concubine Wang circulated. The emperor's anger escalated, and he ordered the execution of the concubines and their relatives. Three thousand people were punished to eradicate any potential enemies.

This created panic among the Imperial Physicians. The situation was so drastic that the head of the Ministry of Health went to Nanjing to seek advice from his former superior, Lord Liu Chun. Lord Liu explained that a physician cannot rely solely on formulae from books passed down from generation to generation. One must consider the evidence and scientific proof in addition to information previously documented.

Lord Liu explained that he and his researchers were testing 5,611 drugs. He had discovered that two harmful herbs, xi xin (细辛) and fu zi (附子), were contained in the traditional formula of ma huang xi xin fi zi decoction (麻黄细辛附子汤) and the si ni decoction (四逆汤), which had been used to treat Concubine Wane. This highlights the importance of finding concrete evidence to prevent further mishaps because traditional formulae may not always be reliable or appropriate.

There are many examples of treatment using traditional prescriptions that contain harmful ingredients.

An empress could not bear children. The imperial physician applied a formula from the tenth century Song dynasty called fu nu yang xue pill (妇女养血丸). This was thought to be a pill for nourishing blood in women. After three years with no success, the imperial physician was executed. During this period, no one thought to analyze the contents of the pill. Reviewing the formula, Lord Liu Chun found that it contained a toxic substance, *Folium artemisiae argyi* (艾叶).

An empress dowager suffered from hysteroptosia (prolapsed uterus) (子宫下垂). The imperial physician applied a traditional formula from the tenth century Song dynasty known as zi bu da li wan (滋补大力丸), and the old queen passed away a few days after ingesting the concoction. Lord Liu Chun later found that it contained copper, frankincense (乳香), and myrrh (没药), all poisonous substances.

A seignior (藩王) suffered from liver problems, and the physician gave him medicine using a formula from the twelfth century Yuan dynasty, long dan xie gan wan (龙胆泻肝丸). The seignior died after six months of treatment, and the imperial physician was executed. The medication contained an poisonous herb, mu tong (木通).

A grandson of the emperor had no appetite, and the physician treated him with a tenth century Song dynasty formula, fei er wan (肥儿丸). After a few days, the grandson's symptoms worsened, and the emperor removed the imperial physician from the post. Lord Liu Chun discovered that the formula contained a harmful herb, rou dou kou (肉豆蔻).

In addition to discovering these harmful elements in the traditional medicines the imperial physicians used, Lord Liu Chun identified herbs that could be harmful to a developing fetus.

Lord Liu Chun's List of Herbs that Cause Cleft Lip

Herb Name	Chinese Name
bai tou weng	白头翁
she gan	射干
qing hao	青蒿
bai zhi	白芷
shi jun zi	使君子

Lord Liu Chun's List of Herbs that Cause Retardation

Herb Name	Chinese Name
hu huang lian	胡黄连
bai jie zi	白芥子
yu xing cao	鱼腥草
rou dou kou	肉豆蔻
hou ma ren	火麻仁
lei wan	雷丸
qian nian jian	千年健

Lord Liu Chun's List of Herbs that Result in Miscarriages

Herb Name	Chinese Name
xing ren	杏仁
ban xia	半夏
wu zhu yu	吴茱萸
jie geng	桔梗

While performing his research in 1410, Lord Liu discovered that many remedies in popular use were derived from documentation of traditional experiences; none of the medicine had been subjected to scientific testing. Lord Liu spent over sixty years researching each of the 5,611 herbs, minerals, and animal products known in traditional Chinese methods. He subjected each item to vigorous testing and conducted many trials to find the effectiveness of each remedy.

To perform a series of four experiments, Lord Liu gathered twenty people:

1. In the first experiment, Lord Liu mixed a specific herb with congee made from millet (第一步，把药材粉末拌入小米粥里让犯人吃), and the patients drank the congee.
2. In the second experiment, Lord Liu ground the medicinal mixture into a powder and added the powder to the patients' bathwater (第二步，把药材粉末放在水里让犯人浸泡).
3. In the third experiment, he burned the medicinal mixture and instructed the patient to inhale the fumes (第三步，把药材粉末燃烧让犯人呼吸).
4. In the fourth experiment, the patients ingested the medicinal mixture with the hunger-inducing soup (第四步，把药材粉末与北山楂，广木香共煮让犯人喝).

Lord Liu adopted an exhaustive trial and error method to identify the best cure for a variety of illnesses. In one case, Lord Liu tested alternative methods of reducing fever. He administered a patient an herb to lower the patient's body temperature. The patient took this herb until experiencing chills, and subsequently, Lord Liu gave the patient an array of herbs to identify the substance that would increase body temperature. In this way, the most efficient herbs for cooling and heating were found. We now understand that, according to modern science, fever patients experience chills not because their body temperature is low but because it is elevated.

Lord Liu Chun commented, "Many people think that this research is cumbersome and a waste of time (是药皆试，或以为愚，非也，莫以流言为是，必欲亲知). These trials must be done because the properties of each ingredient must be known. Performing this research makes me very tired and pressured, however, I will persist until completion (以囚试药力者，其浩繁非比，余衰于此矣)."

He spent sixty-six years on his analysis of 5,611 herbs and food and found 132 of them to be extremely poisonous and not applicable to any cure. He found 911 herbs to be chronically poisonous; these herbs could be used in small quantities or for brief periods, after which they could cause a patient's death. Ingredients in this category include opium and gypsum. Lord Liu found that 4,124 herbs were not effective but were still used. He discovered that 301 foods can be used as medicine and considered 143 of the herbs effective.

In his analysis, Lord Liu Chun discovered also that some herbs could boost the effectiveness of other herbs when the herbs were combined. Lord Liu Chun formulated his family recipes after completing his analysis of the 5,611 herbs and food.

Despite Lord Liu's discovery that some herbs and animal byproducts are ineffective, modern practitioners of Chinese medicine still prescribe a majority of them. In many cases, these ingredients are derived from species that are endangered or rapidly approaching extinction. Medicine that is more effective, less toxic, and less taxing on nature could easily replace bones from tigers and leopards, ivory from elephants, birds' nests, bezoars (牛黄) from cows and monkeys, and other animal byproducts.

The tables that follow list the main ingredients of eighteen Liu family formulae and the ailment that each formula treats.

Liu Family Formula for Treating High Blood Pressure, Stroke, and Coronary Blockage: Tong Xuan San (通玄散)

Ingredients		
Rhizoma Gastrodiae	tian ma	天麻
Common *Macrocarpium* fruit	shan yu rou	山萸肉
Flos Campsis	ling xiao hua	凌霄花
Stigma Croci	xi hong hua	西红花
Rhizoma Polygonati	huang jing	黄精

Liu Family Formula for Treating Asthma and Bronchitis: Na Qi San (纳气散)

Ingredients		
Bulbus Fritillariae Cirrhosae	chuan bei mu	川贝母
Fruit Calyx Seu Fructus Physalis	jin deng long	锦灯笼

Lignum Santali Albi	tan xiang	檀香
Lignum Aquilariae Resinatum	chen xiang	沉香
Colla Cornus Cervi	lu jiao jiao	鹿角胶

Liu Family Formula for Treating Acute Inflammation Including Appendicitis: Ping Chuang San （平疮散）

Ingredients		
Bufo Bufo Gargarizans (Cantor powder)	shao gan chan	烧干蟾
Galla Chinesis	wu bei zi	五倍子
Rhizoma Coptidis	huang lian	黄连
Aloe	lu hui	芦荟
Corydalis turtschaninovii Bess	yuan hu	元胡

Liu Family Formula for Treating Infertility and Erectile Dysfunction: Fu Lao San （扶劳散）

Ingredients		
Radix Angelicae Sinensis	dang gui	当归
Cornu Cervi Pantotrichum	lu rong	鹿茸
Stigma Croci	xi hong hua	西红花
Resina Draconis	xue jie	血竭
Ganoderma Lucidum	ling zhi	灵芝

Liu Family Formula for Treating Cholera, Gastroenteritis, and Diarrhea: Bei Ji San （备急散）

Ingredients		
Rhizoma Coptidis	huang lian	黄连
Fructus Chaenomelis	mu gua	木瓜
Ambergris	long yan xiang	龙涎香
Corydalis turtschaninovii Bess	yuan hu	元胡
Sargentodoxa Cuneata	hong teng	红藤

Liu Family Formula for Treating Pachydermic Cachexia, Asthenic Bulbar Paralysis, and Sleeping Sickness: Su Jue San （苏厥散）

Ingredients		
Radix Ginseng Rubra	Hong shen	红参
Cordyceps Sinensis	chong cao	虫草
Coxtex Cinnamomi	rou gui	肉桂
Ganoderma Lucidum	ling zhi	灵芝
Radix Ledeboruiellae	fang feng	防风

Liu Family Formula for Treating Maintenance of Good Health: Yang Zheng San (养正散)

Ingredients		
Cornu Cervi Pantotrichum	lu rong	鹿茸
Ganoderma Lucidum	ling zhi	灵芝
Radix Ginseng Rubra	hong shen	红参
Ambergris	long yan xiang	龙涎香
Shark gallbladder	sha yu dan	沙鱼胆

Liu Family Formula for Treating Personality Disorder, Hyperthyroidism, Epilepsy, and Narcotics Abuse: Zhi Mi San (指迷散)

Ingredients		
Rhizome Gastrodiae	tian ma	天麻
Succinum	hu po	琥珀
Plastrum Testudinis	gui ban	龟板
Ambergris	long yan xiang	龙涎香
Periostracum Serpentis	she tui	蛇蜕

Liu Family Formula for Treating Diabetes: Han Xiao San (函消散)

Ingredients		
Plastrum Testudinis	gui ban	龟板
Carapax Trionycis	ao jia	鳌甲
Isinglass	yu biao	鱼鳔
Freshwater sponge *Spongilla*	zi shao hua	紫稍花
Stigma Croci	xi hong hua	西红花

Liu Family Formula for Treating Chronic Colitis, Duodenitis, and Gastricism: Cheng Li San (承利散)

Ingredients		
Catechins	er cha jiao	儿茶胶
Pericstraoum Cicadae	chan tui	蝉蜕
Cornu Cervi Pantotrichum	lu rong	鹿茸
	huai mo	槐蘑
Stigma Croci	xi hong hua	西红花

Liu Family Formula for Treating Cancer, White plague, Hemorrhoids, and Tuberculosis: Kong Yan San (控岩散)

Ingredients		
Cornu Saigae Tataricae	ling yang jiao	羚羊角
Lignum Aquilariae Resinatum	chen xiang	沉香
Radix Notoginseng	shen san qi	参三七
Shark gallbladder	sha yu dan	沙鱼胆
Stigma Croci	xi hong hua	西红花

Liu Family Formula for Treating Aregenerative Anemia and Endometrorrhagia: An Chong San (安冲散)

Ingredients		
Radix Notoginseng	san qi	三七
Resina Draconis	xue jie	血竭
Flos Sophorae	huai hua	槐花
Cornu Saigae Tataricae	ling yang jiao	羚羊角
Radix Arnebiae or Radix Lithospermi	zi cao	紫草

Liu Family Formula for Treating Bruises, Tumor, Rheumatoid Arthritis, and Lupus Erythematosis: Hua Pi San (化痞散)

Ingredients		
Endothelium Corneum Gigeriae Galli	jing nei jin	鸡内金
Arisaema Cum Bile	dan nan xing	胆南星
Colla Cornus Cervi	lu jiao jiao	鹿角胶

Ligni Dalbergiae Odoriferae or rosewood	jiang xiang	降香
Resina Draconis	xue jie	血竭

Liu Family Formula for Treating Chronic Nephritis, Cardiomyopathy, and Kidney Stone: Feng Shui San (奉水散)

Ingredients		
Rhizoma Alismatis	ze xie	泽泻
Rhizoma Atractylodis Macrocephalae	bai shu	白术
Ambergris	long yan xiang	龙涎香
Carapax Eretmochelydis	dai mao	玳瑁
Human fingernail	ren zhi jia	人指甲

Liu Family Formula for Treating Relieve Pain, Clear Heat, and Cool blood: Kong Yan Tie Bu (控岩贴布）

Ingredients		
Panax Pseudogingseng Wall	shen san qi	参三七
Zanthoxylum	ma hua jiao	麻花椒
Stigma Croci	xi hong hua	西红花
Shark gallbladder	sha yu dan	沙鱼胆
Menthol	bo he bing	薄荷冰
	feng jiao	枫胶
Colophonium	song xiang	松香

Liu Family Formula for Treating Promote Blood Circulation, Remove Blood Stasis, and Relieve Pain: Hua Pi Tie Bu (化痞贴布)

Ingredients		
Panax Pseudoginseng Wall	shen san qi	参三七
Zanthoxylum	ma hua jiao	麻花椒
Arisaema Cum Bile	dan nan xing	胆南星
Radix Clematidis	wei ling xian	威灵仙
LignumDalbergiaeOdoriferae	jiang xiang	降香
Resina Draconis	xue jie	血竭
	feng jiao	枫胶
*Colophonium*松香	song xiang	松香

Liu Family Formula for Treating Hepatitis, Hepatocirrhosis, Malaria, and Venereal Disease: Bian Zhu San (变痊散)

Ingredients		
Fel Ursi	Xiong Dan	熊胆
Fructus Tsaoko	Cao Guo	草果
Contex Mangoliae Officinalis	Hou Pu	厚朴
Rhizoma Alismatis	Ze Xie	泽泻
Fructus Mume	Wu Mei	乌梅

Liu Family Formula for Treating Flu, Acute Tracheitis, SARS, and Pneumonia: He Feng San (和风散)

Ingredients		
Fel Ursi	Xiong Dan	熊胆
Bambusae Concretio Silicae	Tian Zhu Huang	天竹黄
Caragana frutex	Jin Que Hua	金雀花
Cornu Saigae Tataricae	Ling Yang Jiao	羚羊角
Mint	Bo He Ye	薄荷叶

Chapter 10
Further Observations by Lord Liu

Adverse Drug Reactions

In 1442, Empress Zhang (张氏太皇太后) died in Beijing at the age of sixty-three. For failing to cure his royal patient, the imperial physician (Dr. Gao Qi Zhi 高启智) was executed. Dr. Gao had attempted to simultaneously cure her of three illnesses: asthma/bronchitis, coronary heart disease, and osteoporosis. The empress suffered from difficulty in breathing, headaches, chest pains, and insomnia. The imperial physician treated the empress for her respiratory problems in the morning, for osteoporosis in the afternoon, and for her chest pains at night. Her condition worsened, and after a month, she began to cough up blood and lose her appetite.

Dr. Gao immediately sent a messenger to Nanjing to consult with Lord Liu Chun, who declared that the empress's death was imminent.

He recommended that the three-pronged medical treatment be discontinued immediately and urged Dr. Gao to focus on one illness at a time. Lord Liu Chun argued that the other illnesses would be kept in remission through the restoration of the empress's health. Unfortunately for the empress and for Dr. Gao, Lord Liu Chun's remedies were implemented too late, and the royal patient did not recover.

Lord Liu Chun knew the importance of treating one disease at a time because of his various experiments. He once conducted a study on twenty people with severe asthma. He asked soldiers to beat the patients until they were weak and bruised. He then divided them into four trial groups of five each.

- Lord Liu gave the first group pork skin soup; appetite-inducing soup containing bei shan zha, guang mu xiang, sha shen, and gua lou (北山楂, 广木香, 沙参, 瓜蒌); and asthma medicine, na qi san (纳气散). After a month of treatment, the patients were cured of their asthma, but they still suffered from their bruises and open wounds.

- The second group received fish soup; appetite-inducing soup containing bei shan zha, guang mu xiang, fang feng, and chuan xiong (北山楂, 广木香, 防风, 川芎); and medicine to heal the bruising , hua pi san (化瘀散). After a month, the bruises were gone, but the asthma remained.

- Lord Liu gave the third group two different courses in the morning and evening. In the morning, the group consumed appetite-inducing soup (containing bei shan zha, guang mu xiang, sha shen, and gua lou (北山楂, 广木香, 沙参, 瓜蒌); asthma medicine, na qi san (纳气散); and pork skin soup. In the evening, the patients consumed fish soup; a different appetite-inducing soup containing bei shan zha, guang mu xiang, fang feng, and chuan xiong (北山楂, 广木香, 防风, 川芎); and medicine for the bruises (化瘀散). During this trial, Lord Liu Chun tried a different approach to cure the two problems with two different soups and medicines. After a month, all the ailments remained.

- The fourth group received appetite-inducing soup containing bei shan zha, guang mu xiang, sha shen, and gua lou (北山楂, 广木香, 沙参,

瓜蒌); pork skin soup; fish soup; and asthma medicine, na qi san (纳气散). After a month, the patients were cured of asthma, and their bruises and wounds had healed.

Using many different medications for a variety of diseases did not lead to the patient's recovery. This approach resulted in faster deterioration of the patient's health. After repeating this experiment in several trials, Lord Liu Chun documented that the illnesses should be prioritized. Caregivers should treat the most urgent illness with medicine and the remaining ailments with nutrition therapy. For example, if a patient suffered from cancer, diabetes, and rheumatism, Lord Liu Chun would have proposed medicine for the cancer and food therapy (beef, fish, and tendon soup) to treat the other ailments.

In 2001, the US Food and Drug Administration published a report on adverse drug reactions (ADRs). In 2000, the Institute of Medicine estimated that about seven thousand people die annually from pharmaceutical contraindications. This is an alarming figure. In comparison, approximately six thousand people die annually from workplace injuries. Other statistical sources indicate that the number of ADR-related deaths should be closer to a hundred and six thousand. This would propel ADRs to a staggering fourth place on the list of leading causes of death in the United States—ahead of pulmonary disease, diabetes, AIDS, pneumonia, and accidental or automobile-related deaths. These statistics do not even include the ADRs that take place in ambulances or nursing homes. More than three hundred fifty thousand ADRs occur annually in nursing homes. ADRs cost our health care system $136 billion annually—this is more than the cost of cardiovascular or diabetes care in the United States. One-fifth of the deaths of hospitalized patients are due to ADRs.[1]

The FDA has continued to scrutinize the ADR epidemic. Some of the findings include the following:

1. The volume of drugs the medical community is using to treat patients has increased. An estimated 64 percent of all patients who visit the doctor are given a prescription.
2. In 2000, 2.8 billion prescriptions were filled. This is about ten prescriptions per person.
3. The likelihood of ADRs increases exponentially when a patient is prescribed four or more types of medication.[2]

Today, drugs are tested and approved after being used by an average of one thousand five hundred patients over a short trial period. Given such short trials, it is difficult to detect potential negative interaction between pharmaceuticals.[3]

These modern findings reflect Lord Liu Chun's research because they indicate that combining medicine can have adverse affects. He proved that nutritional therapy and the treatment of one illness at a time, starting with the one that is most life-threatening, yielded the most positive effects on the patient.

We welcome scrutiny of our ideas and treatments and encourage more detailed research of the methodology. During any trials, researchers must give serious consideration to Lord Liu's Ten Points to the Enhancement of Life. No amount of treatment can be effective if the patient indulges in a lifestyle that is contraindicative.

Researchers commonly perform pharmaceutical trials on a mixed group of healthy and ailing patients. In order to test the effectiveness of a new medicine, we suggest that the ailing patients be first given a course of appetite-inducing soup to prepare their bodies and make them as receptive as possible to the test medicine.

Static and Magnetic Electricity

In the summer of 1427, twenty soldiers escorted two hundred prisoners to Liaodong on the northeastern border of China. The prisoners had successfully taken part in Lord Liu Chun's research and were being pardoned from their death sentences. They arrived in a small hostel in Shan Dong province at nightfall. The prisoners had walked such a great distance that their shoes had fallen apart. The soldiers were still wearing their boots.

The twenty soldiers were divided into four squadrons of five men each in preparation for the rotational nighttime guard duty. One of the older soldiers rinsed his feet in hot water in a bronze basin. A thunderstorm suddenly broke out, and lightning struck. The soldier claimed that a fiery red ball blazed across the sky and hit the ground. He was too tired, however, to investigate, and he went to bed.

The next morning, the owner of the hostel awakened the soldier and exclaimed that all the soldiers were dead and the prisoners had escaped.

The old soldier took the hostel owner into custody and went to Lord Liu Chun in Nanjing with his report. Lord Liu Chun asked for the release of the owner of the hostel and the pardon of the prisoners. He asked the governor of the province to bury the nineteen fallen soldiers, despite the ancient Chinese belief that being struck by lightning was an evil omen of the gods.

Lord Liu Chun and several other doctors investigated this matter and debated furiously why all but one of the soldiers had been struck by lightning and why the prisoners had survived. The answer to this peculiar case lay in the footwear of the men who had died. All the soldiers who'd died had worn their shoes to bed, or they had been on guard duty with their shoes on. The old soldier alone had taken off his shoes to wash his feet, while the prisoners' shoes were all broken or too damaged to be worn.

Over time, Lord Liu Chun postulated that a person *who walked barefoot for at least one hour each day* suffered from far less sickness than those who did not.

Lord Liu Chun developed the idea that the yang energy of the human body needed to be balanced with the yin energy of the earth

（人之阳气必与地气接通。不然易遭雷劈，亦发怪病）. Otherwise, the excess yang energy would attract electrical energy (lightning), and the patient would be more susceptible to many odd diseases. Lord Liu also recommended that people should exercise barefoot.

In ancient times, acupuncturists who worked in the royal palace would take off their shoes before they began treatment on a patient. It was a common belief that doing so would enable the doctor to more efficiently stimulate the meridians (通经络) of the patient.

Dr. Liu Hong Zhang, a descendant of Lord Liu Chun, once performed a study in a hospital in Lan Zhou that involved two groups of ten dogs.

Researchers placed one group in doghouses with wooden floors. The other group lived in houses with concrete floors. Researchers observed that the first group exhibited unconventional behavior and was unresponsive to calls by the trainer.

The second group, which was housed in the quarters with concrete floors, responded immediately when called and seemed jovial and playful. At the end of each month, researchers weighed the dogs; the second group weighed more despite being fed the same amounts.

After half a year, researchers measured the dogs' brainwaves. The first group of dogs had beta (δ) brainwaves, indicating lethargy. The second group had alpha (α) brainwaves, indicating alertness. Researchers then placed all the dogs in housing with concrete ground.

Incisions made on the dogs' skull bone healed at different rates in the two groups of dogs, with the first group healing more slowly than the second.

After another year of living in the quarters with concrete floors, the first group returned to normal behavior, and there were no apparent differences between the groups.

Western Research

In March 2006, the World Health Organization recognized that much research must be done on the relationship between electromagnetic fields and public health, particularly with respect to the carcinogenicity of static fields and its correlation to cancer.[4]

In 2009, the WHO announced that it would be releasing a study that links cell phone use to an increased risk of brain and salivary gland tumors. This decade-long study claims to have found a definite link, though it stops short of inferring direct causation.[5]

The US Department of Labor has also been probing the health effects of extremely low frequency radiation. On its official Web site, located at www.osha.gov, the US Department of Labor states, "The issue of extremely low frequency (ELF) biological effects is very controversial. Research has focused on possible carcinogenic, reproductive, and neurological effects. Other possible health effects include cardiovascular, brain and behaviour, hormonal and immune system changes."[6]

Other American institutions have performed in-depth investigations on the effects of electricity. In the National Institute of Environmental Health Sciences Working Group Report of August 1998, a majority of experts concluded, "The electric and magnetic fields like those surrounding electric power lines should be regarded as a 'possible human carcinogen.'"[7]

In a fact sheet that the Centers for Disease Control and Prevention (CDC) provided in 2005, the CDC outlined the effects of the radiofrequency field produced by cell phones on health.

When asked whether cell phones cause health problems, the CDC stated, "In the last ten years, hundreds of new research studies have been done to more directly study possible effects of cell phone use."[8] Although some studies have raised concerns, the scientific research, when taken together, does not indicate a significant association between cell phone use and health effects.[9]

In 1993, the London Hazards Centre published a report on the effects of video display units (VDU) on skin. People who were exposed to VDUs found that they had unpleasant skin blemishes, including a red rash on the face, itching, peeling, raised spots or pimples, or glowing sensations like sunburns. A 1992 Swedish study of six hundred people who use VDUs at work observed that people who used the VDUs for four or more hours experienced skin problems twice as easily as those who only used a VDU for an hour or less.[10]

Ergonomic experts have suggested that businesses use antistatic carpets or vinyl tiles in the workplace; they have also recommended the practice of *walking barefoot* at work. Corporations and business owners should also install humidifiers and select chairs containing conductive material. Employees should wear cotton or conductive clothing instead of synthetics, including polyester.[11]

In April 2007, Sweden issued a warning against wearing rubber clogs in hospitals due to the volume of static electricity buildup and its interference with electronic equipment.[12]

A survey performed in China and India in 1949 found that people who had never worn shoes suffered less from onychrocryptosis (ingrown nails), hyperhidrosis (excessive sweating), bromidrosis (foot odor), and hallux valgus (bunions). They were found to have very few foot problems.[13]

In 2006, Dr. Najia Shakoor and Dr. Joel A. Block of Rush Medical College in Chicago performed a study that found that adults suffering from osteoarthritis were aided in recovery by simply *walking around barefoot*. The study, which was published in *Arthritis and Rheumatism*, suggested, "Modern shoes may exacerbate the abnormal biomechanics of lower extremity osteoarthritis."[14]

We welcome scrutiny of our ideas and treatments and encourage more detailed research of the methodology. During any trials of the methodology, volunteers or patients must also apply Lord Liu's Ten Points to the Enhancement of Life. No amount of treatment can be effective if the patient indulges in a lifestyle that is contraindicative.

Research on the side effects of cell phone usage and static electricity from electronic appliances is still inconclusive. We recommend continued studies on this subject using a test group in bare feet. This test group may reveal that walking with bare feet on surfaces that conduct electricity (earth, concrete, ceramic, and stone) allows excess static electricity to safely flow away from the body.

The King of Boni and Alcoholism

In 1405, Imperial Eunuch Zheng He (郑和) was sent to the areas around Malaysia, Melaka, and Indonesia. He was assigned 27,800 soldiers and 317 ships for his diplomatic mission. Eunch Zheng He helped establish a great trading union between the countries. As trade relations improved, many foreign kings visited China.

In 1408, the King of Boni (西洋渤泥国王) and his family visited China. During the visit, the king died suddenly. The king's family accused Emperor Yon Le of assassination. The emperor was furious and immediately called for an inquest into the death. He summoned Lord Liu Chun to court to investigate the circumstances. The Emperor Yong Le had bestowed many gifts upon his royal visitors, and every day, the imperial chefs had prepared a feast of rich food to celebrate their good relations. Lord Liu Chun inspected the king's corpse, which had been laid on a slab of ice to retard decomposition. He did not find any evidence of poison. Imperial Physician Wang Wen Qiu (王文秋) noted that he had given the king a decoction of long dan xie gan tang (龙胆泻肝汤) and prescribed a vegetarian diet.

Lord Liu Chun found no problems with this prescription and called for the king's diplomat/interpreter, Du Xi Liang. After some time, imperial staff members located the diplomat in a brothel.

Lord Liu Chun asked the diplomat what ailments the king had complained of. Du Xi Lian replied that the king had not been seriously ill and seemed healthy after the medicine, even resuming his habit of drinking strong liquor and eating heavy meals. Lord Liu noted that the diplomat was smirking as he completed his report.

Later it came to light that, every night, the king of Boni had visited the brothel. In fact, he had fallen into a coma at the brothel and had been carried back to the palace, where he was declared dead. Lord Liu Chun finished his report on the death of the king and concluded that the king of Boni had suffered from acute hepatitis. Drinking strong liquor further damaged his liver. He had suffered a hepatic coma due to liver failure. The king's skin was yellowish. Imperial Physician Wang's prescription had been correct in attempting to purge the body of intoxication. The nightly excesses had taken a toll on the king's life.

Emperor Yong Le explained the death to the Boni queen. The queen was embarrassed by her husband's habits and accepted Lord Liu's report as the cause of death.

The emperor ordered the execution of his Boni diplomat/ interpreter and had Imperial Physician Wang caned for negligence. Later, the king of Boni was buried in Nanjing, and Emperor Yong Le personally attended the funeral. The emperor gave the queen of Boni many gifts of gold to compensate for the accidental death of her husband.

The Study of Alcohol

When people fall ill, they are quick to seek a medical remedy, but their condition often fails to improve because they continue to consume large quantities of alcoholic beverages.

In 1406, the general Zhu Neng (朱能) died at the age of thirty-seven. At that time he was leading eight hundred thousand soldiers to fight in An Nan. The cause of his death was his heavy drinking of strong liquor. Before the Ming dynasty, distillation had not been invented, and the percentage of alcohol in liquor was low. After the discovery of distillation during the early Ming dynasty, the alcohol content in liquor reached a level of 65 percent.

In 1406, liquor using this distillation method was very expensive and was considered an item of luxury. People of high rank were given distilled alcohol as gifts, and many people, including the general, died.

Lord Liu Chun decided to study the effects of alcohol and selected thirty death row inmates to conduct an experiment.

Participants in the first group were in their twenties; the members of the second group were in their forties, and the last group was in their sixties. None of the subjects consumed alcohol regularly. Every day, they were instructed to drink approximately 500 milliliters, of the 65 percent alcohol. Within one year:

- The first group suffered from memory loss, shortened attention span, and reduced learning ability.
- The second group experienced myocardiosis and chest pains (心肌病)
- The third group had ascites due to cirrhosis and liver problems (肝硬化腹水).

After many trials, Lord Liu Chun concluded that consuming alcoholic beverages is detrimental to health and impairs specific internal organs. The reason for this specific impairment is still unknown today.

Most religions discourage consumption of alcohol; some even forbid it.

Lord Liu Chun forbade his family and his descendents from drinking any alcohol. As a Buddhist and a medical researcher, he was familiar with the negative impact. To this day, the Liu family avoids alcohol even in preparation of food.

In 2008, the University of Toronto published an article entitled, "One Drink of Red Wine or Alcohol is Relaxing to Circulation, but Two Drinks is Stressful." The research defined a drink as four fluid ounces. Lord Liu Chun performed experimentation with beverages containing 65 percent alcohol, but red wine contains only 12 percent alcohol. Modern theory indicates that small quantities of low-percentage alcohol are beneficial to the heart but detrimental to the liver and to patients suffering from cancer or diabetes. There has only been proof for the benefits to the heart. For this reason, Dr. Liu Hong Zhang requires that the patients he treats who suffer from liver disease, cancer, and diabetes strictly avoid alcohol.

Child Raising: From Conception to Maturity

According to Lord Liu Chun, a woman who wants to conceive should eat a diet rich in vegetables. Once she becomes pregnant, she should change her diet to include meat soup and foods high in fiber. This includes millet, corn, buckwheat, barley, chestnuts, and legumes (such as mung beans and red beans). Her diet should also include fruit, fruit juice, and meat or freshwater fish soups. She should avoid fatty foods and carbohydrates as much as possible.

In ancient times, a pregnant woman suffering from morning sickness received the medicine xuan fu dai zhe shi tang (旋复代赭石汤). There were serious side effects, and children were often born with psychological disabilities. Lord Liu observed cattle and found that the pregnant livestock ate a certain wild plant, purslane (马齿苋). After much research and experimentation, Lord Liu found that the stem and leaves could cure a patient of morning sickness. This plant was mixed with meat to form dumplings that would cure the pregnant women of the imperial court of morning sickness. Every day, the women consumed small amounts.

After giving birth, some of the imperial women had difficulty lactating. To aid in this process, Lord Liu gave the women freshwater fish soup. After experimenting with the dosage, Lord Liu was surprised to find that the best and most effective fish soups were made from small amounts of smaller fish (about six fish, which weighed two taels each, about one pound in total of fish). Additionally, he gave the women bovine Achilles tendon soup to replace the nutrients they lost during pregnancy. He also instructed the women to breastfeed in a sitting position.

Parents can give babies broth made from turnips and bei shan zha. The broth increases babies' metabolism and stimulates their "stomach energy." The following is the recipe for a single serving.

Turnip Broth

50 grams turnip, sliced

50 grams Hawthorn berries

1/2 liter cold water

(1) Soak the turnip and Hawthorn berries in water for thirty minutes.
(2) Drain.
(3) Add half a liter of water, and place the mixture in a glass pot. Bring to a boil and reduce heat. Simmer for 30 minutes.
(4) Strain the turnip and berries, retaining only the liquid. Place the broth in an insulated container to retain the heat. Do not sweeten.

Give the child fifty milliliters each day; the mother should drink the remainder. You can administer dosages three or four times daily. Add the broth to fresh apple juice for improved taste.

According to Lord Liu Chun, caregivers can give a one-month-old baby a broth made from one hundred grams of eggshell boiled in the mixture of turnip and bei shan zha. This increases the soup's calcium content, as the calcium in the eggshell dissolves in the boiling, acidic soup.

At three months, the baby can drink turnip and bei shan zha broth with added bovine Achilles tendon soup for collagen.

At six months, he or she can eat a rice porridge (congee) made of rice, water, pork, or beef liver.

Since the fontanel on the baby's skull has not fully hardened, the child should sleep on a pillow that is made of cao jue ming (*cassia tora L*草决明), the ripe seed of the sicklepod plant. Soy beans are too large, green beans are too round, and rice is too small; the recommended seed is the right size. Use three pounds of cao jue ming to form a pillow with a thickness of about a centimeter. Because the baby always likes to look at his or her mother, it is easy for the baby to sleep only on one side. It is advisable for the mother to sleep on alternating left and right sides of the baby to rotate the baby's head.

Lord Liu recommends that parents and caregivers assign children chores to do at home. This will instill in them a sense of family and responsibility, as well as to prevent them from becoming lazy and dependent on others. Children should learn how to cook, care for their clothes, and be a working member of the family.

Children should be lively and joyful. They should be able to communicate with people of all ages. Parents and caregivers should also teach them courtesy and respect. Caregivers should reprimand a child who has misbehaved in private, in order to preserve his or her dignity. Children should remember their childhood as a positive, happy experience.

Dr. Liu Hong Zhang recalled a personal experience with his father. One day, an important guest visited the Liu household, and the future Dr. Liu was being mischievous. He kept blowing in the guest's ear. His father apologized to the guest but did not scold the child immediately. After the guest had departed, Dr. Liu's father took his son aside and simply explained to him that blowing into someone's ear would cause the person to become deaf. The doctor did not confront his child about the rude behavior; he only explained to his son that his behavior was wrong and asked him not to repeat it again.

When Dr. Liu was a child, he was not shy and could deliver speeches in front of hundreds of people without being nervous. The disciplinary style of the Liu family echoes the teachings of Lord Liu Chun. Children are treated with respect and not reprimanded in public.

Children should do physical exercise. At about a month after birth, parents should help their baby stretch his or her arms and legs. At one to two years old, the child should begin to do sit-ups. At three to four years old, the child should run and jump rope. At ages four to five, the child should work on his or her grabbing power, wrist movement, and leg strength. Most importantly, the child should learn many ball sports. From six to seven years of age and onward, the child should learn self-defense and weightlifting.

Caregivers should encourage children to study and be prepared for school. Children should look over school material before teachers present the material in class, so that they can ask thoughtful questions and absorb the material more quickly.

Caregivers should teach children to respect people and nature. They should feel kindness toward animals and refrain from violence toward any living thing.

Children should have hobbies. This is the foundation for living a life with passion. Hobbies create a healthy outlet for stress and reduce the likelihood of depression and suicide in adulthood. Hobbies include gardening, art, collecting, music, and sports. They must be mentally and physically stimulating and require dedication and commitment.

Activities such as watching movies and shopping for clothes are not hobbies. In the United States, the third leading cause of death in people from the age of ten to twenty-four is suicide. As of 2003, suicide was ranked after motor vehicle accidents and homicide on the list.[15] From early on in life, children should learn motivation in life through developing hobbies and interests.

Parents should take time to have meaningful conversations with their children, encourage their curiosity, and help them learn about the world.

Parents should expose their children to the world of faith and religion. In 2006, a survey concluded that more than 80 percent of the world's population is religious. Practicing a religion can instill a sense of belonging, stability, and tranquility. Every religion encompasses ideas regarding nature, love, life, kindness, charity, service, self-discipline, morale, happiness, spirituality, destiny, truth, death, prayer, friendship, duty, humility, honesty, knowledge, wisdom, bravery, family, compassion, good will, and marriage.

Children should drink meat soup and fresh fruit juices six times a day. Furthermore, they should eat vegetables and food containing high fiber twice a day to provide a healthy and balanced diet. A child's body should be strong and lean.

The Liu family chooses its leader based upon the candidate's health. None of the successors are overweight because soft, cherubic people tend to be of lethargic body and mind (肥头大耳，败家蠢儿). Our current fast-paced lifestyle and obsession with being slim has resulted in a diet laden with carbohydrates, additives, and artificial flavoring. These foods are unhealthy for human consumption and are detrimental to the health of a growing child.

Caregivers should encourage children to play with blocks, building toys, and sand or water toys. Through these, they can learn to value simplicity. Many complicated structures and ideas have simple roots. Children can learn that, by starting with a small object, they can construct something larger and more complex.

Children can also learn the importance of logic through these types of toys. The construction of block structures and the manipulation of sand or water toys stimulate a child's visual and sensory perception. These activities improve the child's ability to estimate measurements of length, weight, volume, and direction.

Caregivers should discourage children should from computer games, especially portable, handheld devices. Although proponents would argue that computer games improve motor skills and reflexes, computer games result in more harm than good. Repetitive, jerky movements stress and overstimulate the body and mind. Computer games discourage social skills, creativity, and interpersonal cooperation. The child becomes a robotic extension of the electronic device and loses contact with the natural world around him or her.

While Dr. Liu Hong Zhang was chief of staff at a Western medical hospital in China, he challenged his staff with a problem. He asked his team of doctors to guess how much an unmarked container could contain. These highly trained professionals guessed volumes ranging from a few milliliters to several thousand milliliters. This presented a very troublesome revelation; the medical staff did not have the visual and analytical skills to estimate the volume in a container. Without measuring devices to guide them, they would not be able to guess how much vital fluid a patient had lost and when the fluid loss would be critical.

Caregivers should give young people thoughtful guidance on different aspects of life as they reach puberty. This is the age at which it is easiest for a person to learn bad habits. It is the time of greatest change and argument. This is when caregivers must nurture young people.

Lord Liu recommends a soup made of sha shen, cao jue ming (*cassia tora L*), and pig skin soup for young adults during puberty. In the 1960s, a beautiful lady visited the Liu household. Dr. Liu Hong Zhang, then a teenager, reacted by having an erection. The guest was very embarrassed. The teenager spent the rest of the night obsessing over the lady's physique. He dreamed of his future wife touching his genitalia. Dr. Liu Hong Zhang could not stand this feeling and asked his father what to do. His father told him to drink the soup. A month later, he found that his sexual urges were less frequent.

The Liu family, unlike many traditional Chinese families, encouraged their children to marry for love. They valued health, morality, and intelligence in the selection of a partner. Despite the Liu family's status as imperial physicians, they did not despise those who were uncultured, unemployed, or underprivileged. In *Your Lifestyle is the Cause of Disease* (2006, 459), Dr. Liu Hong Zhang mentions that his son was considering marriage, the best families in China brought their daughters to meet him. The son, however, had fallen in love with a farmer's daughter.

The farmer did not approve of the match. He said to Dr. Liu, "You are a descendant of a famous doctor, Liu Wan Zhu. Why does your son wish to marry a farmer?"

Dr. Liu replied, "In front of Buddha, everything is equal."

The farmer still disapproved. "My daughter is uneducated."

The doctor responded, "Marriage is not about school or books; it is about life."

The farmer persisted. "My family is very poor."

Dr. Liu Hong Zhang said, "A wealthy man might not be a gentleman. A poor man might not be uneducated. The most important thing is that a person be hardworking and kind."

The farmer finally agreed, and the couple was married. The most important thing in marriage is love. Wealth and power are far less important than building a relationship based upon love and mutual respect.

This collection of child raising tips is compiled from the personal experience and public experiments of the Liu household. The Liu family adheres to a list of thirty-six points on child raising, and we have presented some of the most significant issues in this section. Raising a child can be difficult, and the Liu family urges parents to exercise patience.

Some Unique Chinese Methods for Identifying Illness

Hippocrates has been revered as the father of Western medicine. He was among the few practitioners of his time to recognize symptoms and form a medical diagnosis based on his observations. As a result, Hippocrates was able to identify and classify many medical terms such as Hippocratic face, Hippocratic fingers, and Hippocratic succession. The health care community has also named methods that Hippocrates pioneered after the great Greek physician; these include the Hippocratic bench and the Hippocratic cap-shaped bandage.[16]

Lord Liu Chun also relied on the power of observation in his analyses. In addition to traditional methods of diagnosis (see "Traditional Methods of Diagnosis" at end of chapter), Lord Liu Chun found the following indicators of illness six centuries ago:

1. Lack of hunger

    The feeling of hunger is a direct indicator of the functioning of the body's metabolism and the absorption of nutrients through food. If hunger is not present, sickness is imminent.

    Chronic diseases, like cancer, can be predicted in their earlier stages, as patients who suffer from such diseases are often found to have a lack of hunger a few months prior to official diagnosis.

2. Athlete's foot without itchiness

   If a person suffers from athlete's foot (脚癣) but the affected area does not feel itchy, this is a sign of poor health. In this case, the lack of an itchy feeling would suggest that the nervous system is not functioning properly.

3. Pimples without pus

   Lord Liu Chun could determine if cancer patients had malignant tumors by using garlic. He would rub raw garlic onto a person's forehead to create inflammation. If a pimple with yellow pus (黄脓) developed, the patient did not have cancer. On the other hand, a pimple without pus would point to the possibility of cancer because pus is the result of the body's immune system responding to infection. Dr. Liu Hong Zhang has observed that many cancer patients did not have pus on inflamed areas several years before they were diagnosed with cancer.

4. Hemorrhoids or hernia

   These can be an indication of collagen deficiency in the body. Lord Liu Chun observed that cancer spreads more rapidly when there is a deficiency of collagen (in other words, when there is nothing to "enclose" or prevent cancerous tumors from spreading).

5. Lord Liu considered sudden growth of dense and long eyebrow hair (浓眉) another indication of cancer.

6. Excessive body heat after perspiration

   Perspiration is the body's method of lowering body temperature. If the skin remains hot after perspiration (肤热), the body's homeostasis is malfunctioning, and the body is no longer regulating its temperature properly.

7. Irregular hormone production

Disease can also be diagnosed from irregular patterns in hormone production. Sexual organs are affected by chronic disease. In males, a symptom of disease is sagging scrotum/testes (阴囊下坠). In females, excessively dry genitalia (clitoris) (阴唇干) is a symptom of chronic disease.

8. Bad circulation

This is another significant cause of chronic disease. Patients with chronic stiff necks and upper backs that cause a hunch or curved back (颈椎和圆背) often exhibit poor circulation.

9. Condition of the outer ear

Traditional Chinese doctors use the ear to cure many diseases and pain because it is believed to represent a canvas of the entire body. Wrinkles on the earlobe represent heart disease (耳珠有折纹).

Careful observation is vital to medical practitioners, especially in the matter of life or death. In 2008, the British *Daily Mail* reported a prime example of the power of observation. When general practitioner Dr. Chris Britt met Mark Guerrieri, they shook hands. Immediately, the doctor felt odd because Mr. Guerrieri's hand felt "fleshy and spongy." Mr. Guerrieri also had "large facial features," which led Dr. Britt to recall the symptoms for acromegaly, a fatal disease originating with a benign brain tumor. The most interesting detail about acromegaly is that, in a million people, only three people will have it. Mr. Guerrieri was diagnosed and treated for acromegaly, and he survives today because of Dr. Britt's attention to detail.

Recognition of symptoms will always have great influence on diagnosis and cure. Practitioners must define and understand the problem before they can implement any solution. Failure to do so might inflict delay and high costs; it might even cost a life.[17]

Traditional Methods of Diagnosis

1. *Inspection* (望诊): Examine the patient's spirit and expression, color of skin and face, excretions, body structures, condition of tongue, and symptom site for swelling, alignment, shape, and sensation.

2. *Auscultation and olfaction* (闻诊): Listen to the sound of the patient's voice, abdominal sounds, breathing, and coughing. Smell.

3. *Inquiry* (问诊): Solicit from the patient general information; family and personal history; current complaints; sleep pattern; bowel movements; urination; appetite and digestion; thirst; nutrition levels; chills and fever; emotional health; sexual activity; condition of skin, hair, nails, and teeth; menstrual cycle, and gynecological symptoms.

4. *Palpation and pulse taking* (切诊): Check the qualities and positions of the right and left radial pulses and evaluate, in comparison with a healthy pulse, the following attributes: the regional pulse site texture, temperature, moisture, and sensitivity. Evaluate the tissue structure of the chest, abdomen, ear, and points along channels of the fourteen meridians.

Chapter 11
Frequently Asked Questions

This section provides a summary of the Liu family's work in an easily accessible format. The brief answers summarize the family's recommendations for specific health-related inquiries.

1. **How do I avoid illness?**

   Promote energy in the stomach and true hunger.

2. **How do I avoid cancer from secondary cigarette smoke?**

   Drink appetite-inducing soup and bovine deep flexor tendon soup or Lord Liu's extraction from bovine bones using a secret herbal recipe (刘家骨胶原粉).

3. **What is the process of retarding cancerous growth?**

   Drink appetite-inducing soup, bovine deep flexor tendon soup, and one of Lord Liu's recipes, kong yan san, which contains shark gallbladder.

4. **How do I treat diabetes?**

   Drink appetite-inducing soup, pork or beef skin soup, and Lord Liu's recipe, han xiao san, which contains tortoise shell.

5. **How should doctors treat a person with multiple diseases?**

Identify the most life-threatening ailment and cure it first. Instruct patients to drink one type of appetite-inducing soup, take only one type of medicine to cure one disease at a time, and practice food therapy to nourish the body and avoid adverse drug reactions.

6. **What is the key to the enhancement of life?**

Hunger. (Recent discoveries of hormones affecting hunger,such as leptin, orexins ,ghrelin and obestatin shine additional light on Lord Liu Chun's concept of hunger.)

7. **How do I stimulate my hunger?**

Drink one liter of cold water in the morning. Eat a light dinner. Drink only juice and meat soup. Do abdominal exercises to strengthen the neck muscles. Drink appetite-inducing soup.

8. **What is the worst enemy of a person who is ill?**

No hunger. Traditional Chinese doctors believe that, if there is no energy in the stomach and therefore no hunger, a person will not survive. Life is fueled by energy in the stomach.

9. **What is appetite-inducing soup?**

It is a soup made from one hundred grams of bei shan zha (Hawthorn 北山楂) and fifty grams of guang mu xiang (广木香).

10. **How do I preparing the appetite-inducing soup?**

Appetite-inducing Soup

100 grams bei shan zha

50 grams guang mu xiang

Water for steeping

2 liters fresh water

10 dried red dates (optional)

(1) Place the bei shan zha; guang my xiang; and if desired (to improve the taste), dates in a heat-proof, glass pot. Cover with cold water steep for thirty minutes. Steeping has two benefits: it cleans the herbs and makes boiling easier.

(1) Drain and cover with one liter of fresh water. Bring to boil. Simmer for thirty minutes.

(1) Drain. Add one liter of cold water to the herbs and reboil. Simmer for thirty minutes. Drain into a glass container.

This should produce one and a half liters of soup. Drink in one hundred-milliliter servings at room temperature, preferably finishing the soup within one day. Discard any remaining soup. Do not add any sweetener, sugar, or honey.

For children under the age of four, adults weighing less than 110 pounds, or elderly persons over the age of seventy, reduce the dosage by half.

Cancer patients who are drinking the soup and whose sense of appetite is returning should continue drinking the soup at least every other day.

Once the appetite has stabilized, do not overeat. In the evening, consume only meat soup or fruit juices. Feeling hungry is an important step in the body's return to good health.

11. **If a person has disease, what should he add to the appetite-inducing soup?**

If a person has cancer, add fifty grams of chrysanthemum (杭菊花) and fifty grams of zhu ling (朱苓).

If a person has high blood pressure or circulatory ailments (such as heart problems or stroke), add fifty grams of sha shen (沙参) and twenty grams of chuan xiong (川芎).

12. **Why should cancer patients not eat seafood?**

According to Lord Liu Chun, seafood contains iodine, which dissolves phlegm and tumors. This will lead to the metastasis of cancer cells.

13. **If a person is weak, how can he recover his strength the most effectively?**

Drink fish soup made from freshwater fish or minced beef soup that has been simmered slowly for twelve hours.

14. **Many herbs contain pollutants or are counterfeit. How can one find good quality herbal medicines?**

Look for a reliable and honest herbal medicine shop that has been in the community for years and has regular clientele.

15. **Are there any Western remedies derived from traditional herbal medicines?**

There are many, such as aspirin, which was made from the bark and leaves of willow trees.

16. **What was Lord Liu Chun's view on human experimentation?**

Six hundred years ago, the emperor ordered Lord Liu Chun to perform these experiments. Despite Lord Liu Chun's belief that the most effective cure would be developed through human testing, he felt that it was morally wrong. He performed his experiments on death row inmates with the stipulation that the emperor would be asked to spare the lives of those who survived the experimentation. As a result, hundreds of thousands of death row inmates were saved from death.

17. |**Is human experimentation currently being performed?**

Yes, and it is highly regulated by internationally accepted standards such as the Nuremberg Code.

18. **Have any large-scale human experiments been performed recently?**

The US Department of Defense (DOD) performed mass human experimentation involving hundreds of thousands of military personnel. The department received severe criticism over the matter in a 1994 report entitled "Is Military Research Hazardous to Veteran's Health? Lessons Spanning Half a Century." The paper documented the result of a Senate report that John D. Rockefeller IV chaired. The Web site listed in the references can provide more information.[1]

Chapter 12
Lord Liu at the End of His Days

In 1435, Emperor Xuan De (宣德皇帝) died at the age of thirty-eight. He had consumed Taoist elixirs, which he believed would lead to personal transcendence and eternal life. Instead, he suffered lead poisoning.

In 1487, Emperor Cheng Hua (成化皇帝) followed a course of elixirs prescribed by the Taoists and died of lead poisoning at the age of forty.

Lord Liu Chun analyzed the early demise of these Ming emperors. He made three observations:

1. The emperors were served elixirs three times a day—in the morning, afternoon, and night. These elixirs contained mercury and lead, as well as other toxins.
2. The emperors did little or no physical exercise. Even walking was limited because they were transported in palanquins and bathed by their servants.
3. Every night, the emperors were encouraged to have intercourse with the empress or imperial concubines to increase the number of future heirs.

Lord Liu Chun noticed that only one Ming emperor, Zhu Yun Wen (皇帝朱允文), who was overthrown by his own uncle, Emperor Yong Le (朱棣), lived for a long time and died at the age of ninety-four.

Lord Liu Chun came up with six explanations for this emperor's longevity:

1. Emperor Zhu Yun Wen did not consume the elixirs prepared by the Taoists.
2. He ate simple foods.
3. He performed his own activities and chores.
4. He became a monk, thereby eschewing the complications and stress of court life for days of serenity and spirituality.
5. He was open-minded and content with his life. He did not harbor any regrets or grudges against his uncle who terminated his reign.
6. He enjoyed art and nature, expressing his joy through poetry.

In 1467, Lord Liu Chun presented the results of his experiments to the emperor, but he received no reply. At the time, the emperor favored the Taoists. Emperor Cheng Hua (成化皇帝) invited thousands of Taoists to assemble in Beijing, giving them high salaries and a high status. The emperor believed that their elixirs could increase his sexual ability and ultimately lead to eternal life. The emperor was convinced that Taoists had cures for all illnesses and that, as alchemists, they could transform soil into gold. Imperial physicians, at times, were obliged to listen to the Taoists, who had no medical background. Even in the justice system, court officials would often be forced to yield to the Taoists, who would determine the final verdict!

After several years without any comments on his research from the emperor, Lord Liu Chun decided to retire in 1475. He instructed a faithful servant to hire an old Taoist to inspect his chambers and declare that the energy in the chambers was very negative and that death would befall the occupants within a hundred days (杀气太重，百日之内，必有血光之灾). Lord Liu pretended to be alarmed when he received the news and immediately implored the emperor to terminate his commission and release the three hundred imperial physicians and researchers. He also arranged for one final act of kindness. Lord Liu pardoned the last five thousand death row prisoners and had them sent to Liao Dong in northeastern China to live the rest of their lives as free men.

Lord Liu returned to his hometown in Xianning, Hebei, where he wrote twenty volumes containing sixty-six years of research— *Cheng Hua Xian Ning Jing Hou Jia Xue* (成化咸宁景厚家学). His descendants, who cherish these volumes, have safeguarded them and passed them down through many generations. Lord Liu also instructed his descendants to continue the family tradition of medical service with integrity, honesty, and skill.

Of the twenty volumes, seven contain information regarding cancer. The twenty-fourth descendant of Lord Liu Chun, Dr. Liu Hong Zhang, has stated that he has released less than 10 percent of all the research documented by his famous ancestor to preserve the family secrets. There is still much more information in the volumes that could benefit modern researchers.

In 1475, Lord Liu Chun, then 112 years old, had already spent sixty-six years researching and identifying cures for numerous diseases. The research had spanned the reigns of seven emperors, who did not dare to question the mandate of their royal predecessor. Therefore, Lord Liu Chun's sixty-six years of research, supported by the government and substantiated by hundreds of thousands of tests on death row inmates, was unique both in the medical history of China and in that of the world.

In 1488, the imperial court in Beijing summoned Lord Liu Chun's great-grandson, Liu Wei (刘谓), to become an imperial physician. Liu Wei tried to add some Taoist chemical elixirs into Lord Liu Chun's recipes. Lord Liu Chun was outraged and ordered his servants to give his own son, Liu Jing (刘憬), forty lashes for the actions of his grandson. Lord Liu's son, Liu Jing, survived the lashes. He was 108 years old at the time.

According to the Liu family tradition, the role of the clan elder does not always pass from father to son. Instead, the grandfather chooses an heir from among his grandsons. Liu Jing was punished because he had been responsible for selecting Liu Wei.

After this incident, Lord Liu Chun fell ill, and in September 1489, he died at the age of 126.

When Liu Wei returned to his hometown to attend Lord Liu's funeral, he received eighty lashes. In front of Lord Liu Chun's coffin, his newly written book containing the Taoist alchemy methods was burned.

Upon the death of Lord Liu, the Emperor and all high-ranking officials sent their condolences to the family. Because Lord Liu was a fervent Buddhist, he wanted a simple burial. At his grave, there is not even a tombstone; only bamboo trees were planted. Lord Liu's life was filled with countless acts of selflessness, and his influence upon Chinese medicine is enormous. He lived each day under the light of the Liu family motto: "Do not seek to know one's future, but do good deeds" (但做好事，莫问前程).

Lord Liu was posthumously conferred the title of Patron Saint of the Imperial Physicians of the Ming and Qing dynasties (明清太医保护神).

In 1941, Dr. Liu Lian Zhong (刘连仲) and his two sons were captured during the Japanese occupation of China. Their captors demanded all the books and formulae that Lord Liu Chun had produced. Dr. Liu and his sons refused and were executed. Their bodies were never recovered.

Chapter 13
Imperial Physicians and the
Family Tree of Lord Liu Chun

Nine hundred years ago, Dr. Liu Wansu (刘元素) (1110–1194) was known as the preeminent physician during the Jin and Yuan dynasties (金元朝).

He found that shark gallbladder could be used in the treatment of cancer. He discouraged people from eating fatty foods and carbohydrates in favor of high fiber foods.

One of his most renowned mottos was "Do not seek to know one's future, but do good deeds" (但做好事，莫问前程).

To this day, there stands in the province of Hubei a temple constructed in Liu Wansu's honor for the many lives he saved during an epidemic.

In "A Medical Line of Many Masters: A Prosopographical Study of Liu Wansu and His Disciples from the Jin to the Early Ming," published in *Chinese Science II*, Dr. Wu Yiyi made evident that Dr. Liu Wansu and his students were the first lineage to be recognized in the Siku Quanshu (四库全书) in the sixteenth century Qing dynasty imperial library collection.[1]

Dr. Liu Wansu's ninth-generation descendant was Lord Liu Chun (1363–1489). Lord Liu's medical expertise was so great that he was conferred the title of Patron Saint of Imperial Physicians during the Ming and Qing dynasties (明清太医保护神). This is comparable to the reverence bestowed upon Saint Luke, the Patron Saint of Physicians and Surgeons, in the Christian faith.

Following the emperor's decree, Lord Liu Chun, together with three hundred doctors and several thousands of soldiers, spent sixty-six years conducting experiments on hundreds of thousands of death row inmates to identify the cure for many diseases.

He developed Ten Points to the Enhancement of Life (养生十法), a guideline to preventing illness.

Mr. Nathan Sivin, professor of Chinese culture at the University of Pennsylvania, authored of an article entitled "Science and Medicine in Chinese History." Sivin stated that, until recent times, Chinese medicine was only available to the upper class of the social hierarchy in China and that the majority of the Chinese population had limited access to qualified physicians.

The majority of China's patients and more eminent practitioners belonged to the upper crust of society. Over the course of history, most of the afflicted among the Chinese population had no access to the small number of qualified physicians. They depended on a great variety of less educated healers, ranging from herbalists to priests—a situation comparable to that existing in eighteenth-century France.

What we call "medicine" incorporated and imposed order on experiences related to every aspect of health, disease, and injury. One Chinese scheme of major divisions includes theoretical studies of health and disorder; therapeutics; the theory and practice of longevity techniques, including sexual hygiene; pharmacognosy; and veterinary medicine.

Pharmacognosy, the study of vegetable, animal, and mineral substances used in therapy, brought together so much information on the sources and characteristics of thousands of drug ingredients that its literature was studied not only for therapeutic purposes, but also as compendia of natural history.[2]

During the Ming dynasty, the Tai Yi Yuan (太医院)—similar to the Ministry of Health—had two functions. Its primary function was to take care of the health of the royal family, and secondarily, it was to manage all government hospitals. The ministry had thirteen divisions: internal medicine, pediatrics, wind-caused disease, obstetrics, ophthalmology, stomatology, dentistry, pharyngolaryngology, bone setting, miscellaneous diseases, acupuncture, moxibustion, and prayer healing and incantation.

During the Qing dynasty, the ministry added a smallpox division (天花科) was and intermittently recognized acupuncture as a division.

Lord Liu Chun was the head of this ministry. When the imperial court relocated to the Forbidden City in Beijing, Lord Liu remained in Nanjing to continue his research to identify the cure for many diseases.

Following in the footsteps of Lord Liu Chun, twelve of his descendants were appointed imperial physicians and served the emperor. Most of the others were appointed to positions in the imperial medical bureau. Following their ancestor's philosophies of life and nutrition, they all exceeded normal life expectancy. The following table outlines Lord Liu Chun's descendants.

Lord Liu Chun's Descendants

Rank 辈次	Name	Birth	Death	Age	Occupations
Tai Zu 太祖	Liu Wan Su 刘完素	1110	1194	84	Preeminent physician in the Jin and Yuan dynasties
Gao Zu 高祖	Liu Chun 刘纯	1363	1489	126	Minister of health, Patron Saint of Imperial Physicians
Descendent 1 承袭1	Liu Jing 刘憬	1381	1496	115	Vice minister of health
Descendent 2 承袭2	Liu Yu 刘宇	1404	1495	91	Vice minister in Shanxi province

Descendent 3 承袭3	Liu Wei 刘谓	1436	1527	91	Imperial physician
Descendent 4 承袭4	Liu Kan 刘刊	1463	1549	86	Imperial physician
Descendent 5 承袭5	Liu Lang 刘琅	1489	1579	90	Director of Ministry of Health
Descendent 6 承袭6	Liu Yi 刘镒	1513	1597	84	Director of Ministry of Health
Descendent 7 承袭7	Liu Qiang 刘檣	1539	1631	92	Director of Ministry of Health
Descendent 8 承袭8	Liu Duo 刘沰	1562	1669	107	Minister of health
Descendent 9 承袭9	Liu Ye 刘烨	1590	1681	91	Minister of justice
Descendent 10 承袭10	Liu Shang 刘墒	1619	1708	89	Chief of imperial pharmaceutical factory
Descendent 11 承袭11	Liu Yun Sheng 刘允生	1641	1678	37	Chief of imperial pharmaceutical factory
Descendent 12 承袭12	Liu Gao Pu 刘高普	1659	1750	91	Chief of imperial pharmaceutical factory
Descendent 13 承袭13	Liu Xiang Xian 刘相贤	1692	1784	92	Chief of imperial pharmaceutical factory
Descendent 14 承袭14	Liu Liang Yu 刘良玉	1712	1803	91	Imperial physician
Descendent 15 承袭15	Liu Jian Xun 刘见巽	1736	1807	71	Chief of imperial pharmaceutical factory
Descendent 16 承袭16	Liu You Tang 刘佑堂	1761	1842	81	Chief of imperial pharmaceutical factory
Descendent 17 承袭17	Liu Hou Ru 刘厚如	1782	1873	91	Chief of imperial pharmaceutical factory
Descendent 18 承袭18	Liu You Wei 刘由卫	1803	1903	100	Chief of imperial pharmaceutical factory

Descendent 19 承袭19	Liu Qi Hou 刘启后	1825	1911	86	Imperial physician
Descendent 20 承袭20	Liu Xuan Ji 刘璇玑	1851	1939	88	Imperial physician
Descendent 21 承袭21	Liu Lian Zhong 刘连仲	1873	1941	68	Physician to President Yuan Shi Kai
Descendent 22 承袭22	Liu Feng Chi 刘凤池	1897	1948	51	Physician to President Jie Shi Jiang
Descendent 23 承袭23	Liu Shi Kui 刘世奎	1922	1991	69	Medical doctor
Descendent 24 承袭24	Liu Hong Zhang 刘弘章	1946			Medical doctor, Head of the Liu family as of this writing
Descendent 25 承袭25	Liu Bo 刘渤	1977			Medical doctor

Lord Liu Chun's eleventh descendant, Liu Yun Sheng, lived to be only thirty-seven years old. He sold medicine that the family had not authorized, and his own relatives buried him alive.

Lord Liu Chun's twenty-first descendant, Liu Lian Zhong, died when he was sixty-eight years old. The Japanese executed him and two of his sons for refusing to divulge the family formulae. The American ambassador to China, John Stuart (司徒雷登大使), was a close friend of Liu Lian Zhong. He tried to save his friend but was unsuccessful. After World War II, Mr. Stuart brought Lian Zhong's sixth son to America. In 1967, this son offered the therapeutic results of 5,611 herbs studied by Lord Liu Chun to the Food and Drug Administration in New York.

Corrupt officials betrayed Lord Liu Chun's twenty-second descendant, Liu Feng Chi, and he was murdered in prison at the age of fifty-one.

There are more than ten thousand Liu family members globally. As of this writing, the head of the family is Dr. Liu Hong Zhang in Tianjin, China.

Liu Chun's Mottos

- Do not seek to know one's future, but do good deeds (但做好事, 莫问前程).
- Medication provides no cure when a patient loses his hunger and desire to live (有胃气则生, 无胃气则死).
- A good physician tastes the medicine to be provided to his patient (药不亲尝不发).
- A person has himself to blame for neglecting his own health (病是自家生).
- Seventy percent of life is sustained through constant maintenance of good health (nurturing), and thirty percent by reliance on good medicine (healing) (七分养, 三分治).
- A faithful follower of Buddha gains peace of mind; with peace of mind, he lives to his heart's content, thereby freeing himself from anger. He is constantly blessed with happiness that, in turn, prevents illness. Thus Buddha is the ultimate physician. To faithfully believe in Buddha is one way to keep one's mind in harmony in order to secure a state of juvenescent health (信佛而通达, 通达而知足, 知足而不恼, 不恼而常乐, 常乐而不病, 故佛乃上工。).
- One depends on one's hunger and desire to live. Without these, life comes to an end (无胃气, 不知饥者, 则死).

Chapter 14
Conclusion

When Dr. Liu Hong Zhang began to write about the research of Lord Liu Chun, many family members voiced their disapproval. They did not wish to disclose the family secrets, particularly to the Chinese people. Dr. Liu's grandfather had worked for the Taiwanese government during the Second Sino-Japanese war and Dr. Liu's father had suffered during the Cultural Revolution under the communist regime.

Nevertheless, Dr. Liu pursued his vision to share the family's wealth of knowledge, and he completed the three books that recount a tenth of the research and experiences of Lord Liu Chun.

Dr. Liu extended his dedication to sharing alternative medical methods when he heard that the current supply of bovine deep flexor tendon in China is limited or of poor quality. Dr. Liu has begun the process of extracting type I collagen from pig and cow bones by replicating one of the secret recipes of his famous ancestor.

Three years after the publication of Dr. Liu's books—*Lord Liu Chun's Enhancement of Life*, which links food therapy and healthy living to the prevention of many diseases; *Your Lifestyle is the Cause of Disease*, which details the effects of certain lifestyles that cause disease; and *Beware of Medicine*, which proclaims that medicine can cause new problems, a book published in 2008 corroborated the information and recommended treatments from the earlier books. The author, Zhao Ying Jian (赵英健), is a noted Communist television director whose team contacted 119 people in twenty-three provinces to discuss their experiences with Dr. Liu. Many of the interview subjects cited other friends or family members who had followed Dr. Liu's treatment so that, in actuality, more than 1,000 people were documented in the study. The interview subjects represented a full spectrum of society—farmers, pilots, teachers, entrepreneurs, monks, Western medical doctors, and academicians—and ranged in age from infants to octogenarians. They suffered from illnesses including cancer, diabetes, hepatitis, cardiovascular disease, hypothyroidism, renal lithiasis, and uremia.

After following the initial food and hunger therapy segments of Dr. Liu's approach to longevity—*seven parts nurturing, three parts healing*—many of the subjects experienced significant improvement in their condition, while others were fully cured. Mr. Zhao was amazed at the success rate of the treatments. After three months of inquiry, his team had amassed so much positive feedback that they were forced to reject further offers from subjects who had heard about the inquiry and wanted to share their own experiences. Dr. Liu's books were bestsellers in China and caused a tremendous interest in food therapy. The treatment for cancer using bovine deep flexor tendon was so popular that it led to a shortage in the supply in several Chinese provinces. Similarly, the herb used in the preparation of appetite-inducing soup, guang mu xiang, became scarce due to interest in this treatment.

One particular documented case was that of Professor Qi Jian Xun (乞建勋). The team leader of mathematical research in China (NPC=NP research), Professor Qi was a renowned for solving an important classic mathematical problem.

At sixty-two years old, Professor Qi discovered in April 2007 that he suffered from kidney cancer. Three of China's best oncology hospitals confirmed his condition. He decided to implement Dr. Liu's natural approach to illness because, as a scientist himself, he believed that the human body was a system, and illness could only be prevented if the immune system was functioning properly and the body was in equilibrium. Because his own mother and wife had adopted Dr. Liu's *seven parts nurturing* with success, Professor Qi decided that Dr. Liu's treatment of cancer would provide the most health benefit with the least interruption to his important research.

After a year of treatment, Professor Qi reported that his cancer was in remission, his blood pressure had been reduced, and he no longer suffered from high cholesterol. He believed that his current health was better than it was ten years earlier. Like many other subjects interviewed, Professor Qi made his own identity known so that he could share his experience and lend credibility to the Liu family approach.

Another case involves a well-known professor of information technology, Professor Wang Yong Cheng (王永成). Academician of the Chinese Academy of Sciences and the European Academy of Sciences Institute of Arts and Humanities, he had received more than nine years of traditional Western medical treatment for his diabetes, with little success. In 2006, his doctors had advised his family to prepare for the worst because his health had severely deteriorated. As a last resort, Professor Wang followed the treatment for diabetes suggested in Dr. Liu's books by preparing daily portions of pig skin soup. Being a scientist himself, Professor Wang agreed to regular monitoring of his glucose level, cholesterol, and blood pressure.

After three months of pig skin soup, Professor Wang's glucose level was reduced by 300 percent. His doctor initially claimed that this would only be a short-term improvement, but Professor Wang had maintained his healthy glucose level for two years as of this writing. This case aroused the interest of the hospital's dietician, who launched a study of the benefits of pig skin therapy.

Dr. Liu's books have significantly impacted people from all walks of life. In a remote and impoverished village of Shanxi province (陜

西省), villagers have become accustomed to yearly flu resulting in the death of many children. After adopting the methods from Dr. Liu's book on the enhancement of life, there have been fewer severe cases of flu and no further flu-related deaths.

Friends and students of Dr. Liu have worked hard for the past two and a half years to translate, edit, and correlate modern medical research with Lord Liu's research.

Despite the medieval concepts of feudalism, morality, and corporal punishment prevailing in his time, Lord Liu Chun requested the return to good health and release of the prisoners upon their completion of the experiments. Although hundreds of thousands of people were freed, hundreds of death row inmates also died in the process.

Bibliography

REFERENCES CITED

Ahmet, Ismayil, Ruiqian Wan, Mark p. Mattson, Edward G. Lakatta, and Mark Talan, "Cardioprotection by Intermittent Fasting in Rats," (American Heart Association, 2005), http://circ.ahajournals.org/cgi/content/abstract/112/20/3115.

Akre, Jane, "WHO Warns of Long-term Cell Phone Risk," *InjuryBoard.com* (2009), http://www.injuryboard.com/national-news/who-warns-of-longterm-cell-phone-risk-.aspx?googleid=273368.

AllExperts, Lorry, "Computer Security & Viruses," AllExperts (2005), http://en.allexperts.com/q/Computer-Security-Viruses-1737/virus-57.htm.

American Cancer Society, "Poor Appetite," American Cancer Society (2008), http://www.cancer.org/docroot/MBC/content/MBC_6_2X_Poor_Appetite.asp?sitearea=MBC

Bakalar, Nicholas, "Regular Midday Snoozes Tied to a Healthier Heart," *The New York Times* (February 13, 2007), http://www.nytimes.com/2007/02/13/health/13nap.html?ref=health.

BBC News, "Fibre 'Lowers Breast Cancer Risk'," (2007), http://news.bbc.co.uk/go/pr/fr/-/2/hi/health/6287915.stm.

BBC News, "Frequent Sex 'Not Linked to Strokes,'" BBC News Online (2002), http://news.bbc.co.uk/2/low/health/1763627.stm.

BBC News, "Warm Feet Mean Swift Sleep," BBC Online Network (1999), http://news.bbc.co.uk/2/hi/science/nature/435342.stm.

Bear, Soaring, researcher, "Hawthorn," HerbMed, (Herbmed, 1998, updated 2006 by J Mohanasundaram, researcher), http://www.herbmed.org/Herbs/Herb97.htm.

Bhargava, Pankaj, John L. Marshall, William Dahut, Naiyer Rizvi, Nina Trocky, Jon I. Williams, Howard Hait, Sharon Song, Kenneth J. Holroyd, and Michael J. Hawkins, "A Phase 1 and Pharmacokinetic Study of Squalamine, a Novel Antiagiogenic Agent, in Patients with Advanced Cancers," *Clinical Cancer Research* (2001, 2007), http://clincancerres.aacrjournals.org/cgi/content/abstract/7/12/3912.

Brahmavamso, Ajahn, "The Time and Place for Eating," UrbanDharma.org (Buddhist Society of Western Australia, 1990), http://www.urbandharma.org/udharma3/eating.html.

Brem, Henry, "Squalamine Slows Tumor Growth," *Health Newsfeed* (1998).

Brunel, J. M., C. Salmi, C. Loncle, N. Vidal, and Y. Letourneux, "Squalamine: A Polyvalent Drug of the Future?" abstract, *Current Cancer Drug Targets* 5(4) (2005), http://www.ncbi.nlm.nih.gov/pubmed/15975047

Cameron, James D., Christopher J. Bulpitt, Elisabete S. Pinto, and Chakravarthi Rajkumar "The Aging of Elastic and Muscular Arteries: A Comparison of Diabetic and NonDiabetic Subjects," *Diabetes Care* 26 (2003), http://care.diabetesjournals.org/cgi/content/abstract/26/7/2133

CBS News, "Weight Training Reverses Aging Damage in Muscles: Study," CBC News (2007), http://www.cbc.ca/health/story/2007/05/22/muscle-aging.html.

Centers for Medicare and Medicaid Services, Office of the Actuary, National Health Statistics Group, "National Health Care Expenditures Data," "Historical," 2010, http://www.cms.gov/NationalHealthExpendData/02_NationalHealthAccountsHistorical.asp#TopOfPage.

Chen, Wenhua and Robert Moellering, "A Bioconjugate Approach toward Squalamine Mimics: Insight into the Mechanism of Biological Action," ACS Publications (2006, 2007), http://pubs.acs.org/cgi-bin/abstract.cgi/bcches/2006/17/i06/abs/bc060220n.html.

Chernova, Marina N., David H. Vandorpe, Jeffrey S. Clark, Jon I. Williams, Michael A. Zasloff, Lianwei Jiang, and Seth L. Alper, "Apparent Receptor-mediated Activation of Ca^{2+}-Dependent Conductive Cl-Transport by Shark-derived Polyaminosterols," *The American Journal of Regulatory, Integrative, and Comparative Physiology* (2005), http://ajpregu.physiology.org/cgi/content/abstract/289/6/R1644.

Department of Health and Human Services, "Frequently Asked Questions about Cell Phones and Your Health," Department of Health and Human Services Center for Disease Control and Prevention (2005), http://www.cdc.gov/nceh/radiation/factsheets/cellphone_facts.pdf.

Donohue, B., A. Miller, M. Beisecker, D. Houser, R. Valdez, S. Tiller, and T. Taymar, "Effects of Brief Yoga Exercises and Motivational Preparatory Interventions in Distance Runners: Results of a Controlled Trial," abstract, *British Journal of Sports Medicine* 40 (2006), http://bjsm.bmj.com/cgi/content/abstract/40/1/60.

Eat Right Montana, "Moving Away from Diets: Why and How," *mt.gov* (Montana Department of Public Health and Human Resources, May 1, 2007), http://www.dphhs.mt.gov/newsevents/newsreleases2007/may/awayfromdiets.shtml.

Einstein, Albert to J. S. Switzer, April 23, 1953, *Einstein Archive* 61–381, quoted in Ralph Dumaine, "Albert Einstein on the Secrets of Western Science," *The Autodidact Project* (2000), http://www.autodidactproject.org/quote/einstn2.html.

English, P. and G. Williams, "Hyperglycaemic Crises and Lactic Acidosis in Diabetes Mellitus," abstract, *Postgraduate Medical Journal* 80 (2004), http://pmj.bmj.com/cgi/content/abstract/80/943/253.

Falini, Giuseppe, Simona Fermani, Elisabetta Foresti, Bruna Parma, Katia Rubini, Maria Chiara Sidoti, and Norberto Roveri, "Films of Self-assembled Purely Helical Type 1 Collagen Molecules," abstract, *Journal of Materials Chemistry* 14, (2004), www.rsc.org/publishing/journals/JM/article. asp?doi=b401393j.

Farnsworth. Norman R., "Screening Plants for New Medicines," National Academy Press (1998) www.ciesin.columbia.edu/docs/002-256c/002-256c.html.

Felding-Habermann, Brunhilde, Timothy E. O'Toole, Jeffrey W. Smith, Emilia Fransvea, Zaverio M. Ruggeri, Mark H. Ginsberg, Paul E. Hughes, Nisar Pampori, Sanford J. Shattil, and Alan Saven, "Integrin Activation Controls Metastasis in Human Breast Cancer," abstract, *Proceedings of the National Academy of Sciences of the United States of America* 98 (2001), www.pnas. org/cgi/content/full/98/4/1853.

Floraleads, "Hawthorn," (2008), http://floraleads.com/hawthorn.htm.

Guardian.co.uk, "Plastic Clogs Disrupt Machinery in Swedish Hospital," Guardian.co.uk (2007) www.guardian.co.uk/print/0,,329784836-103681,00.html.

Gilfoy, Christine, contact, "Lungs Try to Repair Damaged Elastic Fibers," American Physiological Society (2006), www.eurekalert.org/pub_releases/2006-11/aps-ltt103106.php.

Gold Bamboo, "Oral Type 1 Collagen for Relieving Scleroderma," Gold Bamboo (2005), http://goldbamboo.com/topic-a117166.html.

Graham, P. A., I. E. Maskell, J. M. Rawlings, A. S. Nash, and P. J. Markwell, "Influence of a High Fibre Diet on Glycaemic Control and Quality of Life in Dogs with Diabetes Mellitus," *Journal of Small Animal Practice*, (2007), http://www.blackwell-synergy.com/doi/abs/10.1111/j.1748-5827.2002. tb00031.x.

Hara, Takako, "Hunger and Eating," California State University (1997), http://www.csun.edu/~vcpsy00h/students/hunger.htm.

Helm, Hughes M., Judith C. Hays, Elizabeth P. Flint, Harold G. Koenig, and Dan G. Blazer, "Does Private Religious Activity Prolong Survival? A Six-Year Follow-up Study of 3,851 Older Adults," Abstract, *Journals of Gerontology* Series A 55(7) (1999), http://biomedgerontology.oxfordjournals.org/content/55/7/M400.abstract.

Herbst, Roy S., Lisa A. Hammond, David P. Carbone, Hai T. Tran, Kenneth J. Holroyd, Avinash Desai, Jon I. Williams, B. Nebiyou Bekele, Howard Hait, and Victoria Allgood, "A Phase I/IIA Trial of Continuous Five-Day Infusion of Squalamine Lactate (MSI-1256F) Plus Carboplatin and Paclitaxel in Patients with Advanced Non-Small Cell Lung Cancer," abstract *Clinical Cancer Research* (2003), http://clincancerres.aacrjournals.org/cgi/content/abstract/9/11/4108?maxtoshow=&HITS=10&hits=10&RESULT FORMAT=&titleabstract=a+phase+1%2F11A+trial+of+continuous+five-day+infusion+of+squalamine+lactate%28MSI-12&searchid=1&FIRSTIND EX=0&resourcetype=HWCIT.

Herlyn, Meenhard, Martin Padarathsingh, Lynda Chin, Mary Hendrix, Dorothea Becker, Mark Nelson, Yves DeClerck, James McCarthy, and Suresh Mohla,

"New Approaches to the Biology of Melanoma: A Workshop of the National Institutes of Health Pathology B Study Section," *American Journal of Pathology* 161 (2002), http://ajp.amjpathol.org/cgi/content/full/161/5/1949.

Hidaka, Muneaki, Ken-ichi Fujita, Tetsuya Ogikubo, Keishi Yamasaki, Tomomi Iwakiri, Manabu Okumura, Hirofumi Kodama, and Kazuhiko Arimori, "Potent Inhibition By Star Fruit of Human Cytochrome P450 3A (CYP3A) Activity," abstract, *Drug Metabolism and Disposition* 32(6) (2004), http://dmd.aspetjournals.org/cgi/content/full/32/6/581

Hitti, Miranda, "Exercise Has Type 2 Diabetes Benefits," *WebMD*, (CBS News.com 2007), http://www.cbsnews.com/stories/2007/09/18/health/webmd/main3271441.shtml.

Holmgren, I., "The Nobel Prize in Physiology or Medicine 1934," *Nobel Lectures, Physiology or Medicine 1922–1941*, (Amsterdam: Elseveir Publishing Company, 1965) (Nobelprize.org), http://nobelprize.org/nobel_prizes/medicine/laureates/1934/press.html).

Howard Hughes Medical Institute, "Loss of Arterial Elasticity May Accelerate Heart Disease," Howard Hughes Medical Institute (1998), http://www.hhmi.org/news/keating3.html.

Hsiao. Jerry I.-H., "Patent Protection for Chinese Herbal Medicine Product Invention in Taiwan," abstract, *The Journal of World Intellectual Property* (2007), http://www.blackwell-synergy.com/doi/pdf/10.1111/j.1422-2213.2007.00311.x?cookieSet=1

Humphreys, Susie and K. R. Porter, "Collagen Deposition on a Preformed Grid," *Journal of Morphology* 149 (2005), http://www3.interscience.wiley.com/journal/109918615/abstract.

Institute for Traditional Medicine, "Hawthorn (Crataegus) Food and Medicine in China," (2007), www.itmonline.org/arts/crataegus.htm.

Integra, "BioMend & BioMend Extend Absorbable Collagen Membrane," (Integra Lifesciences Corporation 2006), http://www.integra-ls.com/products/?product=104.

Jackson, Donald C., "How a Turtle's Shell Helps It Survive Prolonged Anoxic Acidosis," *News Physiology Science* 15 (2000) http://physiologyonline.physiology.org/cgi/content/abstract/15/4/181.

Kappaelastin.com, "Elastin," kappaelastin.com, http://www.kappaelastin.com/html/elastin.html.

Levy, Andrew, "Restaurant Owner's 'Spongy' Handshake with GP Saves Man's Life after Doctor Recognised Rare Killer Brain Tumour," *Mail Online* (2008), http://www.dailymail.co.uk/news/article-514340/Restaurant-owners-spongy-handshake-GP-saves-mans-life-doctor-recognised-rare-killer-brain-tumour.html.

London Hazards Centre, "Chapter 3 – Skin," *VDU Work and the Hazards to Health* (1993), www.lhc.org.uk/members/pubs/books/vdu/vd03.htm.

Lorenzi, Rossella, "Faith Linked to Lower Blood Pressure,".WordPress.com, (2006, 2008), http://doods.wordpress.com/2006/05/27/faith-linked-to-lower-blood-pressure/

Madden, Kathryn, contact, "Oregon Study Confirms Health Benefits of Cobblestone Walking for Older Adults," Oregon Research Institute (2005), http://www.eurekalert.org/pub_releases/2005-06/ori-osc062905.php.

Mager, Donald E., Ruiqian Wan, Martin Brown, Aiwu Cheng, Przemyslaw Wareski, Darrell R. Abernethy, and Mark P. Mattson, "Caloric Restriction and Intermittent Fasting Alter Spectral Measures of Heart Rate and Blood Pressure Variability in Rats," *The FASEB Journal*, (2006), http://www.fasebj.org/cgi/content/full/20/6/631.

Mason, Pamela, "Food and Medicines," The Pharmaceutical Journal (2002), http://www.pjonline.com/pdf/cpd/pg_20021019_drugfood.pdf.

Mount Sinai Hospital, Mount Sinai School of Medicine, "Study Shows Food Preparation May Play a Bigger Role in Chronic Disease than was Previously Thought," *Science Daily* (2007), http://www.sciencedaily.com/releases/2007/04/070424155559.htm.

Murphy, Amy, "Heart Health Benefits of Walking and Sports in Japan," *Medical News Today*, (2005, MediLexicon International Ltd., 2007), www.medicalnewstoday.com/articles/32709.php.

National Heart, Lung and Blood Institute, "What Is Chronic Obstructive Pulmonary Disease?" Apria Healthcare (2009), http://www.apria.com/channels/1,2748,93-203,00.html.

Nicoloff, G. and S. Baydanoff, "Elastin Peptides as a Marker of the Severity of Vascular Complications in Diabetes Mellitus," summary, Department of Biology and Immunology, University School of Medicine, 5800 Pleven, Bulgaria (1997), http://www.idb.hr/diabetologia/97no3-5.html.

National Cancer Institute, "For Cancer-Related Appetite Loss, Cannabis Is No Better than Placebo," The National Cancer Institute (2006), http://www.cancer.gov/clinicaltrials/results/cannabis0806.

National Cancer Institute, "Questions and Answers about Cartilage (Bovine and Shark)," National Cancer Institute (2009), http://www.cancer.gov/cancertopics/pdq/cam/cartilage/patient/40.cdr#Section_40.

New World Encyclopedia, "Hippocrates," (2009), http://www.newworldencyclopedia.org/entry/Hippocrates.

Okumura, Kazuo, Yutaka Nakamura, Seiji Takeuchi, Isao Kato, Yoshinori Fujimoto, and Nobuo Ikekawa, "Formal Synthesis of Squalamine from Desmosterol," *Chemical and Pharmaceutical Bulletin: The Pharmaceutical Society of Japan* 51 (2003), www.jstage.jst.go.jp/article/cpb/51/10/51_1177/_article/-char/en.

Oliwenstein, Lori, "USC Researches Show How Collagen Inhibits Cancer," University of Southern California (2005) (2007), http://uscnews.usc.edu/hscweekly/detail.php?recordnum=11898.

Pache, Mona, Kurt Krauchi, Christian Cajochen, Anna Wirz-Justice, Barbara Dubler, Josef Flammer, and Hedwig J. Kaiser, "Cold Feet and Prolonged Sleep-onset Latency in Vasospastic Syndrome," *Lancet* 358 (2001), http://cat.inist.fr/?aModele=afficheN&cpsidt=1053972.

Pandian, Essakky G., "Pharmacological Evaluation of the Root Powder of Saussurea lappa (Costus)," abstract, (OpenMED@NIC 2006) http://openmed.nic. in/1471/.

Partenheimer, David, "Religious Faith and Spirituality May Help People Recover from Abuse," American Psychological Association (2000), http:// www.scienceblog.com/community/older/2000/A/200000651.html.

Patent Storm, "US Patent 6147060 – Treatment of Carcinomas Using Squalamine in Combination with Other Anti-cancer Agents," abstract, PatentStorm (2000), www.patentstorm.us/patents/6147060.html.

Penniston, Kristina, "Citric Acid and Kidney Stones," *UW Hospital Metabolic Stone Clinic*, (University of Wisconsin 2005) http://www.uwhealth.org/files/ uwhealth/docs/pdf/kidney_citric_acid.pdf.

Pietras, Richard J. and Olga K. Weinberg, "Evidence-based Complementary and Alternative Medicine," *Oxford Journals* (2005), http://ecam.oxfordjournals. org/cgi/content/full/2/1/49.

Piloto, Connie, contact, "Keep Kidney Stones Away with Orange Juice, Not Lemonade," *Medical News Today*, (MediLexicon Internal Ltd. 2006), www. medicalnewstoday.com/articles/50980.php.

King's College London, Public Relations Department, "New Drugs Potential of Chinese Herbs" (2007), http://www.kcl.ac.uk/news/news_details. php?year=2007&news_id=505.

Rangwani, Shanti B., "The Miracles of Fasting: Dr. Shanti B. Rangwani Writes on the Therapeautic Benefits of Fasting," *Islamic Voice* 12:144 (1998).

Ruvini, Liyanage, Naoto Hashimoto, Kyu-Ho Han, Teppei Kajiura, Shoko Watanabe, Ken-ichiro Shimada, Mitsuo Sekikawa, Kiyoshi Ohba and Michihiro Fukushima, "Some Bovine Proteins Behave as Dietary Fibres and Reduce Serum Lipid in Rats," abstract, *British Journal of Nutrition* 97 898–905 (2007), http://journals.cambridge.org/action/displayFulltext?type= 1&fid=986596&jid=BJN&volumeId=97&issueId=05&aid=986588.

Science Daily, "Frequent Sex Linked with Good Health for 70 And 80 Years Olds," Science Daily (2007), http://www.sciencedaily.com/releases/2007/08/070822184023.htm.

Science Daily, "The Power of Fruit Juice," (Science Daily 2007), http://www. sciencedaily.com/releases/2007/09/070905175237.htm

Sinha, S. R. Guleria, A. Misra, R. M. Pandey, R. Yadav, and S. Tiwari, "Pulmonary Functions in Patients with Type 2 Diabetes Mellitus & Correlation with Anthropometry & Microvascular Complications," *The Indian Journal of Medical Research* 119(2), (2004), http://www.ncbi.nlm.nih.gov/ pubmed/15055485.

Sivin, Nathan. "Science and Medicine in Chinese History," (2003, 2007), http:// ccat.sas.upenn.edu/~nsivin/ropp.html.

Skin Health News Editor, "Celebrex Treats Skin Cancer, Shark Bile and Acne," *Health Diaries* (2004), http://www.healthdiaries.com/news/skin/archives/ skin_cancer/celebrex_treats_skin_cancer_shark_bile_and_acne.html.

Smith, Morgan, "Going Barefoot is Good for the Sole," Sports Chiropractic and Massage (2007), http://sportschirodecatur.com/Articles/WalkingBarefoot. htm.

Smith, Stephanie, "Experts Disagree on Ideal Time of Day to Exercise: Doctor Says Late Afternoon Works Best for Body," *CNN.com* (2004), http://www. cnn.com/2003/HEALTH/diet.fitness/05/27/exercise.time/index.html.

Society for Barefoot Living, "Bare Feet and OSHA," Society for Barefoot Living (2006), www.barefooters.org/osha.html.

Starcher, Barry, Ronnie L. Aycock, and Charles H. Hill, "Multiple Roles for Elastic Fibers in the Skin," *Journal of Histochemistry and Cytochemistry* 52 (2005) http://www.jhc.org/cgi/content/abstract/53/4/431.

Stibich, Mark, "Hara Hachi Bu – Eat Until 80 Percent Full," About.com (June 5, 2007), http://longevity.about.com/od/longevitylegends/g/hara_hachi_ bu.htm.

Stump, Amy L., Terri Mayo, and Alan Blum "Management of Grapefruit-Drug Interactions," *American Family Physician* (The American Academy of Family Physicians 2006), www.aafp.org/afp/20060815/605.html.

Sugahara,Takuya, Masashi Ueno, Yoko Goto, Ryusuke Shiraishi, Mikiharu Dio, Koichi Akiyama, and Satoshi Yamauchi, "Immunostimulation Effect of Jellyfish Collagen," Japan Society for *Bioscience, Biotechnology, and Biochemistry* 70 (2006), http://www.jstage.jst.go.jp/article/bbb/70/9/70_2131/_ article.

Suicide.org, "Suicide Statistics," Suicide.org: Suicide Prevention, Awareness, and Support, http://www.suicide.org/suicide-statistics.html.

Sun Media, "Lose Big Time with High Fibre," CHealth, (MediResource, Inc. 2003), http://chealth.canoe.ca/columns.asp?columnistid=1&articleid=6218 &relation_id=3224.

Thompson, Tommy, quoted in "The Prevention Plan," U.S. Preventitive Medicine, http://www.uspreventivemedicine.com/Home.aspx.

Tribole, Evelyn and Elyse Resch, "What's Intuitive Eating?" *Intuitive Eating*, (intuitiveEating.org 2007) http://www.intuitiveeating.com/.

United States Department of Labor, "Extremely Low Frequency (ELF) Radiation: Health Effects," United States Department of Labor Occupational Safety & Health Administration, www.osha.gov/SLTC/elfradiation/healtheffects.html.

United States Food and Drug Administration, "Preventable Adverse Drug Reactions: A Focus on Drug Interactions," FDA (2001).

University of Iowa Health Care, "Why You Should Drink More Water," (University of Iowa Hospitals & Clinics 2006), www.uihealthcare.com/topics/ generalheatlth/ghea5288.html.

University of Maryland Medical Center, "Hawthorn," (2008), http://www.umm. edu/altmed/articles/hawthorn-000256.htm.

US Congress, "Is Military Research Hazardous to Veterans' Health? Lessons Spanning Half a Century," *Storming Media* (Washington, DC, 1994).

Wendel, D. P., D. G. Taylor D, K. H. Albertine, M. T. Keating, and D. Y. Li, "Impaired Distal Airway Development in Mice Lacking Elastin," *American Journal of Respiratory Cell and Molecular Biology* 23(3) (2000) http://www.ncbi.nlm.nih.gov/pubmed/10970822

Williams, John I., Steven Weitman, Cristina M. Gonzalez, Carita H. Jundt, Jennifer Marty, Stephanie D. Stringer, Kenneth J. Holroyd, Michael P. McLane, Qiming Chen, Michael Zasloff, and Daniel D. Von Hoff, "Squalamine Treatment of Human Tumors in *nu/nu* Mice Enhances Platinum-based Chemotherapies·" *Clinical Cancer Research* (2001, 2007). http://clincancerres.aacrjournals.org/cgi/content/full/7/3/724.

Will-Harris, Daniel, ed., "Scientific Proof Confirms Napping Enhances Worker Productivity," eFuse (2000), http://www.efuse.com/nap/.

Winer, N. and J. Sowers, "Diabetes and Arterial Stiffening," M. E. Safar and E. D. Frohlich, editors, abstract, *Artherosclerosis, Large Arteries and Cardiovascular Risk, Advanced Cardiology* 44 (2007), http://content.karger.com/ProdukteDB/produkte.asp?Doi=96745.

World Health Organization, "Electromagnetic Fields and Public Health: Static Electric and Magnetic Fields," (2006), http://www.who.int/mediacentre/factsheets/fs299/en/print.html.

World Wildlife Fund, "Use of Plants for Medicine around the World" (2008).

Yee-Lean Lee, Thomas Cesario, Yang Wang, Edward Shanbrom, and Lauri Thrupp, "Antibacterial Activity of Vegetables and Juices," *Nutrition* 19(11) (2003): 994–996.

Yiyi, Wu. "A Medical Line of Many Masters: A Prosopographical Study of Liu Wansu and His Disciples from the Jin to the Early Ming," *Chinese Science* 11 (1993–94), http://www.uni-tuebingen.de/uni/ans/eastm/back/cs11/cs11-3-wu.pdf.

Yosiaki, Sasazawa, "Afternoon Exercise Improves the Quality of Night Sleep: A Case Study Observed by EEC and Self-Rating Scale," abstract, *Journal of Occupational Health* 40 (1998), http://joh.med.uoeh-u.ac.jp/e/E/40/E40_1_06.html.

ADDITIONAL REFERENCES

Angell, Deborah L., "Eating Disorders Awareness: Binge Eating Disorder," Ohio State University FactSheet, Ohio State Universtiy (2001), http://ohioline.osu.edu/ed-fact/1004.html.

Anson, Michael, Zhihong Guo, Rafael de Cabo, Titilola Iyun, Michelle Rios, Adrienne Hagepanos, Donald K. Ingram, Mark A. Lane, and Mark P. Mattson, "Intermittent Fasting Dissociates Beneficial Effects of Dietary Restriction on Glucose Metabolism and Neuronal Resistance to Injury from Calorie Intake," *Proceedings of the National Academy of Sciences of the United States of America* (2003), http://www.pnas.org/cgi/content/abstract/100/10/6216.

Bicon Dental Implants, "Resorbable Collagen Plug," Bicon Dental Implants (2004), http://www.bicon.com/product_info/pi_new_RCP.html.

Canadian Cancer Society, "Eat Well, Be Active: What You Can Do," Canadian Cancer Society (2004), http://www.cancer.ca/ccs/internet/publication-list/0,,3172_286016785_281087715_langId-en.html.

China Daily, "Pumpkin Could Hold Key to Diabetes Treatment," China.org.cn (2007), http://www.china.org.cn/english/health/216555.htm.

The Consortium of Academic Health Center, University of Michigan Health System, "Water," *Healing Foods Pyramid*, (2004) http://www.med.umich.edu/umim/food-pyramid/water.htm.

C V Mosby Company, St. Louis, "Liver Diet Is Discovered as Treatment for Anemia," (1936) in *OldAndSold Antiques Digest*, http://www.oldandsold.com/articles32n/health-chats-128.shtml.

Duke Medicine News and Communications, "Study to Explore Whether Weight Training Can Reduce Cardiovascular Risk," Duke University Health System (2004), http://www.dukehealth.org/HealthLibrary/News/8119.

Henriet, Patrick, Zhi-Duan Zhong, Peter C. Brooks, Kenneth I. Weinbert, and Yves A. DeClerck, "Contact with Fibrillar Collagen Inhibits Melanoma Cell Proliferation by Up-regulating p27[KIP1]," *Proceedings of the National Academy of Sciences of the United States* (2000), www.pnas.org/cgi/content/abstract/170290997v1.

Higgins, Rosemary D., Raymond J. Sanders, Yun Yan, Michael Zasloff, and Jon I. Williams, "Squalamine Improves Retinal Neovascularization," *Investigative Ophthalmology and Visual Science* 41, The Association for Research in Vision and Ophthalmology Inc. (2000), www.iovs.org/cgi/content/abstract/41/6/1507

Houghton, A. McGarry, Pablo A Quintero, David L. Perkins, Dale K. Kobayashi, Diane G. Kelley, Luiz A. Marconcini, Robert P. Mecham, Obert M. Senior, and Steven D. Shapiro, "Elastin Fragments Drive Disease Progression in a Murine Model of Emphysema," *Journal of Clinical Investigation* 116(3) (2006), www.jci.org/cgi/content/abstract/JCI25617v1.

Kimball's Biology Pages, "Fighting Cancer with Angiogenesis Inhibitors," (2005), http://users.rcn.com/jkimball.ma.ultranet/BiologyPages/A/Angiogenesis.html,http://www.hopkinsmedicine.org/hnf/hnf_812.HTM.

Kumar, Neeraj, Christopher J. Boes, and Martin A. Samuels., "To the Editor: Liver Therapy in Anemia: A Motion Picture by William P. Murphy," *Journal of the American Society of Hematology* 107(12) (2006), Blood online, http://bloodjournal.hematologylibrary.org/cgi/content/full/107/12/4970?ck=nck.

Kyung, Kyu Hang, and H. P. Flemming, "Antibacterial Activity of Cabbage Juice against Lactic Acid Bacteria," abstract, *Journal of Food Science* 59(1) (1994), http://www.blackwell-synergy.com/doi/abs/10.1111/j.1365-2621.1994.tb06915.x.

McMillan, D. E., "The Microcirculation in Diabetes," *Microcirculation, Enothelium, and Lymphatics* 1(1) (1984), http://www.ncbi.nlm.nih.gov/pubmed/6400426?ordinalpos=1&itool=EntrezSystem2.PEntrez.Pubmed.Pubmed_ResultsPanel.Pubmed_DiscoveryPanel.Pubmed_Discovery_RA.

The Medical News, "Heart Bypass Gets New Source for Replacement Blood Vessels," MedicalNews.Net (2004), www.news-medical.net/print_article.asp?id=6263.

Meschia, M, P. Pifarotti, F. Bernasconi, F. Magatti, D. Riva, and E. Kocjancic, "Porcine Skin Collagen Implants to Prevent Anterior Vaginal Wall Prolapse Recurrence: A Multicenter, Randomized Study," abstract, *Journal of Urology* 177(1) (2007), http://www.ncbi.nlm.nih.gov/pubmed/17162041.

Moore, Karen S., Suzanne Wehrli, Heinrich Roder, Mark Rogers, John N. Forrest, Jr., Donald McCrimmon, and Michael Zasloff, "Squalamine: An Aminosterol Antibiotic from the Shark," National Academy of Sciences (2003) (2008) http://www.pnas.org/cgi/content/abstract/90/4/1354.

Patent Storm, "Regioselective and Stereoselective Oxidation of Fused Ring Systems Useful for the Preparation of Aminosterols," Patent Storm (2005), www.patentstorm.us/patents/6933383.html

Schwartz, Joan, "Research Briefs," *B. U. Bridge*, Boston University (2003), http://www.bu.edu/phpbin/researchbriefs/display.php?id=647.

Stephensen, Charles B., Examining the Effect of a Nutrition Intervention on Immune Function in Healthy Humans: What Do We Mean by Immune Function and Who Is Really Healthy Anyway?" *American Journal of Clinical Nutrition* 74(5) (2001), http://www.ajcn.org/cgi/content/full/74/5/565.

Swartz, Daniel D., Russell A. James, and Stelios T. Andreadis, "Fibrin-based Functional and Implantable Small Diameter Blood Vessels," *American Journal of Physiology – Heart and Circulatory Physiology* (2004), http://ajpheart.physiology.org/cgi/content/abstract/00479.2004v1.

Vardaxis, N. J., T. A. Brans, M. E. Boon, R. W. Kreis, and L. M. Marres, "Confocal Laser Scanning Microscopy of Porcine Skin: Implications for Human Wound Healing Studies," abstract, *Journal of Anatomy* 190(pt. 4) (1997), Anatomical Society of Great Britain and Ireland, http://www.pubmedcentral.nih.gov/articlerender.fcgi?artid=1467644.

Vidal, Bde C., "From Collagen Type 1 Solution to Fibers with a Helical Pattern: A Self-assembly Phenomenon," abstract, *Les Comptes Rendus de l'Académie des sciences* 318(8) (1995)..

Wall, Steven J., Erica Werner, Zena Werb, and Yves A. DeClerck, "Discoidin Domain Receptor 2 Mediates Tumor Cell Cycle Arrest Induced by Fibrillar Collagen," abstract, *The Journal of Biological Chemistry* (2005), http://www.jbc.org/cgi/content/abstract/280/48/40187.

Wrong Diagnosis.com "Causes of Poor Appetite," Wrong Diagnosis.com, http://www.wrongdiagnosis.com/symptoms/poor_appetite/causes.htm.

Zhang, Z., W. K. Ho, Y. Huang, A. E. James, L. W. Lam, and Z. Y. Chen, "Hawthorn fruits Hypolipidemic in Rabbits Fed a High Cholesterol Diet," abstract, *Journal of Nutrition* 132(1) (2002), PubMed.gov, http://www.ncbi.nlm.nih.gov/pubmed/11773500.

沈季铭. 周向东. 周维善 "Formal Synthesis of Squalamine from Methylhyodeoxycholanate," (2006) 北京万方数据股份有限公司 (2007) http://scholar.ilib.cn/A-hxxb200614017.html

Zhang, Zesheng, Walter K. K. Ho, Yu Huang, and Zhen-Yu Chen, "Hypoc-
holesterolemic Activity of Hawthorn Fruit is Mediated by Regulation of
Cholesterol-7α-hydroxylase and Acyl CoA: Cholesterol Acyltransferase,"
Food Research International, 35(9) (2002), http://linkinghub.elsevier.com/
retrieve/pii/S0963996902000996.

Notes

Chapter 1: The Last Request of Empress Yong Le
1. Holmgren, "The Nobel Prize."
2. Centers for Medicare and Medicaid Services, "National Health Expenditure."
3. Thompson, "The Prevention Plan."

Chapter 3: Hunger: The Key to Curing Illness
1. Eat Right Montana, "Moving Away from Diets."
2. Stibich, "Hara Hachi Bu."
3. Tribole and Resch, "What's Intuitive Eating?"
4. Brahmavamso, "The Time and Place for Eating."
6. Rangwani, "Miracles of Fasting."
6. Bear, "Hawthorn."
7. Pandian "Pharmacological evaluation of the root powder of Saussurea lappa,"

Chapter Four: Lord Liu's Ten Steps to the Enhancement of Life
1. University of Iowa, "Water."
2. Ahmet, Wan, Mattson, Lakatta, and Talan, "Cardioprotection by Intermittent Fasting,"
3. Mager, Wan, Brown, Cheng, Wareski, Abernethy, and Mattson, "Caloric Restriction and Intermittent Fasting."
4. BBC News, "Fibre 'lowers breast cancer risk.'"
5. Sun Media, "Lose Big Time."
6. Graham, Maskell, Rawlings, Nash, and Markwell, "Influence of a High Fibre Diet."
7. The Mount Sinai Hospital, "Food Preparation May Play a Bigger Role."
8. Murphy, "Heart Health Benefits of Walking."
9. Madden, "Cobblestone Walking."
10. Bakalar, "Regular Midday Snoozes."
11. Will-Harris, "Napping Enhances Worker Productivity."
12. Science Daily, "The Power of Fruit Juice."

13 Penniston, "Citric Acid and Kidney Stones." See also Piloto, "Keep Kidney Stones Away with Orange Juice."
14 Yosiaki, "Afternoon Exercise Improves the Quality of Night Sleep."
15 Smith, "Ideal Time of Day to Exercise."
16 CBS News, "Weight Training."
17 Hitti, "Exercise Has Type 2 Diabetes Benefits."
18 Donohue, et al., "Brief Yoga Exercises and Motivational Preparatory Interventions."
19 Pache, et al., "Cold Feet."
20   BBC News, "Warm Feet."
21 Helm, et al., "Private Religious Activity?"
22 Partenheimer,"Religious Faith and Spirituality."
23 Rossella, "Faith Linked to Lower Blood Pressure."
24 BBC News, "Frequent Sex."
25 Science Daily, "Frequent Sex for 70 And 80 Years Olds."
26 Association and Register of Colon Hydrotherapists, "Common Questions."

Chapter Five: Cancer Research: Modern Versus Lord Liu Chun

1   Altman, "Sharks May Yield a Potent Weapon."
2   Brem, "Squalamine Slows Tumor Growth."
3   "Bhargava, et al., "Pharmacokinetic Study of Squalamine."
4   Williams, et al., "Squalamine Treatment of Human Tumors."
5   Herbst, et al., "A Phase I/IIA Trial of Continuous Five-Day Infusion."
6   Chen, et al. "A Bioconjugate Approach toward Squalamine Mimics."
7   Okumura, et al., "Formal Synthesis of Squalamine."
8   Patent Storm, "Treatment of Carcinomas Using Squalamine."
9   Skin Health News, "Celebrex Treats Skin Cancer."
10   Brunel, et al, "Squalamine: a Polyvalent Drug."
11   Integra, "BioMend & BioMend."
12   Ruvini, et al., "Some Bovine Proteins Behave as Dietary Fibres."
13   Sugahara, et al, "Immunostimulation Effect of Jellyfish Collagen."
14   Humphreys and Porter, "Collagen Deposition."
15   Falini, et al., "Films of Self-assembled Purely Helical Type 1 Collagen."
16   Herlyn, et al., "New Approaches to the Biology of Melanoma."
17   Ibid.
18   Felding-Habermann, et al., "Integrin Activation Controls Metastasis."
19   "Type I Collagen Gene Suppresses Tumor Growth."
20   Gold Bamboo, "Oral Type 1 Collagen for Relieving Scleroderma."
21   Ibid.
22   Einstein to J. S. Switzer.
23   National Cancer Institute, "Cartilage (Bovine and Shark)."

Chapter Six: Diabetes: Lord Liu's Historical Research Versus Modern Research

1   English, and Williams, "Hyperglycaemic Crises."
2   Jackson, "How a Turtle's Shell Helps It Survive."
3   Kappaelastin.com, "Elastin."
4   Nicoloff and Baydanoff, "Elastin Peptides."
5   Cameron, et al. "Aging of Arteries."
6   Wendel, et al., "Impaired Distal Airway Development."
7   Gilfoy, "Lungs Try to Repair Damaged Elastic Fibers."
8   The National Heart, Lung and Blood Institute, "Chronic Obstructive Pulmonary Disease."
9   Starcher, et al., "Multiple Roles for Elastic Fibers."
10 Howard Hughes Medical Institute, "Loss of Arterial Elasticity."
11 Ibid.

CHAPTER SEVEN: FOOD IS MEDICINE

1   Yee, et al., "Antibacterial Activity of Vegetables and Juices."
2   Hidaka, et al., "Potent Inhibition By Star Fruit,"
3   Stump, et al., "Management of Grapefruit-Drug Interactions."
4   American Cancer Society, "Poor Appetite."
5   "Food Preparation May Play a Bigger Role in Chronic Disease."
6   Holmgren, "The Nobel Prize."
7   Ibid.
8   Ibid.
9   Ibid.

Chapter Nine: Chinese Herbal Medicine

1. Hsiao, "Patent Protection."
2   World Wildlife Fund, "Plants for Medicine around the World."
3   Farnsworth, "Screening Plants for New Medicines."
4   Ibid.
5   King's College London, "New Drugs Potential."

Chapter Ten: Further Observations by Lord Liu

1   FDA, "Preventable Adverse Drug Reactions."
2   Ibid.
3   Ibid.
4   World Health Organization, "Electromagnetic Fields."
5   Akre, "WHO Warns of Long-term Cell Phone Risk."
6   United States Department of Labor, "Extremely Low Frequency (ELF) Radiation."
7   Ibid.

8   Department of Health and Human Services, "Cell Phones and Your Health."

9   Ibid.

10   London Hazards Centre, "Skin."

11   AllExperts, "Computer Security."

12   Guardian.co.uk, "Plastic Clogs Disrupt Machinery."

13   Society for Barefoot Living, "Bare Feet and OSHA."

14   Smith, "Going Barefoot."

15   Suicide.org, "Suicide Statistics."

16   New World Encyclopedia, "Hippocrates."

17   Levy, "Restaurant Owner's 'Spongy' Handshake."

Chapter Eleven: Frequently Asked Questions

1   US Congress, "Is Military Research Hazardous?"

Chapter Thirteen: Imperial Physicians and the Family Tree of Lord Liu Chun

1   Yiyi, "A Medical Line of Many Masters."

2   Sivin, "Science and Medicine in Chinese History."

Photos

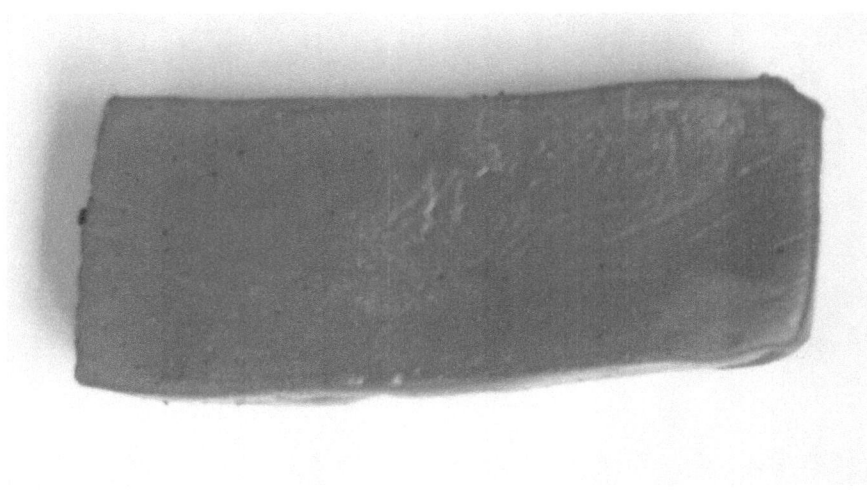

Blood Tofu

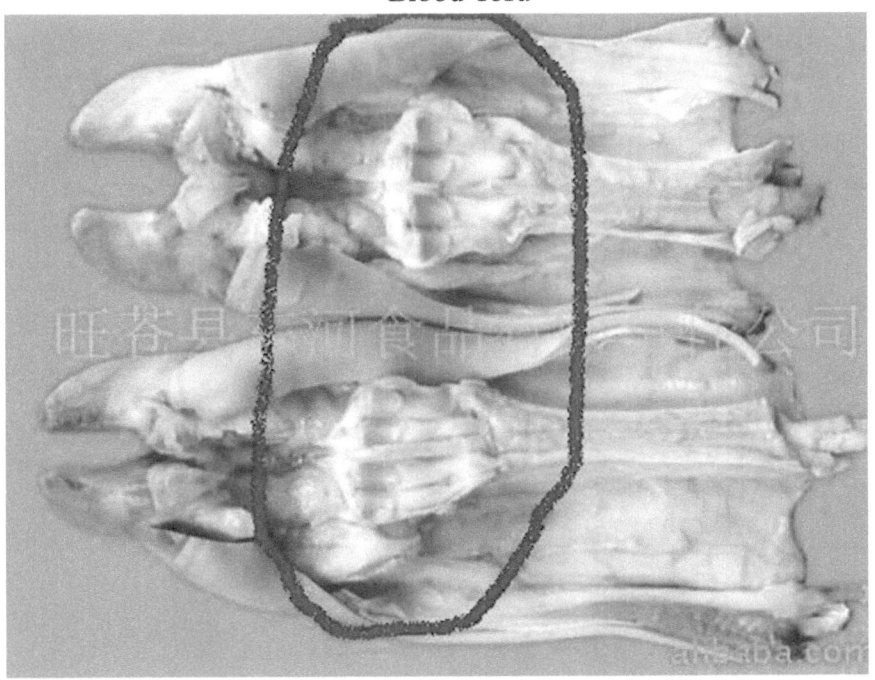

Bovine Flexor Tendon (circled)

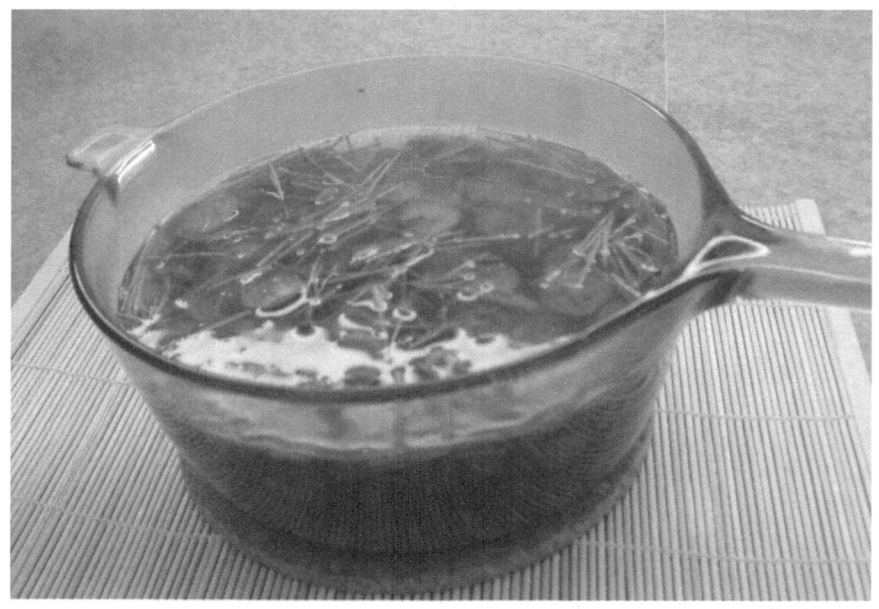

Appetite Inducing Soup

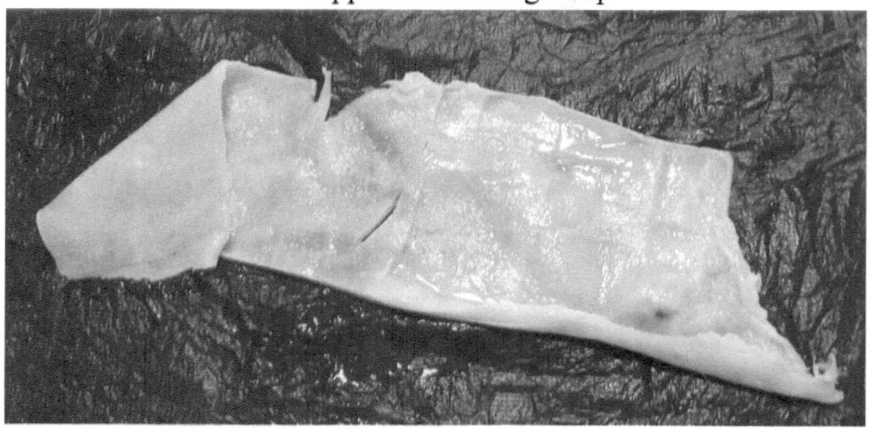

Pig Skin without fat